MY VOICE

A PHYSICIAN'S PERSONAL EXPERIENCE
WITH THROAT CANCER

ITZHAK BROOK, MD

ISBN: 1-4392-6386-8
ISBN-13: 9781439263860

The cover photographs were taken by Yoni Brook

Table of Contents

Dedication

This book is dedicated to my famiiy.

Acknowledgement

The editorial assistance of Autumn Conley is greatly appreciated. I am grateful to my wife Joyce and my son Yoni for their helpful input and advice in writing this book.

Disclaimer

The names of the physicians mentioned in the book were altered.

Introduction

This book captures three years of my life that followed a throat cancer diagnosis and tells my personal story of facing and dealing with medical and surgical treatment and adjusting to life afterwards. This period of my life was and is still very challenging and difficult. As a physician with lifelong experience in caring for patients, I gained realizations, insights and new perspective on these events. I felt for the first time the effects of severe illness through the eyes of a patient and observed and experienced events I was never aware happened to them.

I am sharing my fears, anxieties, frustrations, failures, and ultimate adaptation and adjustment to life with continuous uncertainty about the future. After hearing other head and neck cancer survivors tell their stories, I realized that mine is not unique. It is shared by many others.

It is my hope that the readers of this book will gain insight into the mind of a patient with a life threatening illness such as cancer. I hope this book will assist others in dealing with trying times in their own lives. Most importantly, I hope the book will shed light into the struggles that we face as patients with cancer of the head and neck and how we strive to overcome them. Through my words and my story, it is my hope that physicians, nurses, and other health care professionals may be more aware of what their patients actually experience, and patients who face similar hardships may find out how to cope with them.

Chapter 1. Suspicions

Learning that I had been diagnosed with cancer was overwhelming. It all happened unexpectedly, and I was completely unprepared for it. It all started about three months earlier, and in the most unlikely place.

My throat hurts really badly, I thought, as I lectured to an audience of over 200 Ear and Throat Doctors in Bursa, Turkey. The truth is, my throat was very irritated, and I found that strange because I wasn't otherwise feeling ill at all. As soon as I finished my talk to my colleagues, I went to my hotel room and opened my mouth to see if I could find anything that might explain the pain, but I saw nothing. I rinsed and gargled water, but the pain did not subside.

I was surrounded by hundreds of experienced otolaryngologists but, ironically, I could not ask any of them for help. This was because we were at a beautiful snow resort in the mountains, about 200 miles away from Istanbul, for the Annual Meeting of the Turkish Society of Otolaryngology. They had invited me to give several lectures on head and neck infections. Most of the participating otolaryngologists there were with their families, enjoying the break from their busy lives by skiing and partaking of other resort activities once they had followed the protocol of their scientific agendas. I knew many of the doctors personally. As a physician and an infectious diseases specialist with special interest in head and neck infections for the past decade, I had been here to Turkey to lecture almost annually.

I did mention my symptoms to one of participants, and he offered to examine me in his clinic after the meeting, but I elected to wait and see if the irritating feeling would just go away with time. I decided to wait patiently until I returned to Washington DC, where I could be examined by my own otolaryngologist, Dr. Morell, the Head of the Otolaryngology Department at the Navy hospital in Bethesda, Maryland, where I also worked.

I had collaborated with Dr. Morell, his predecessors, and other residents and staff physicians for over twenty-six years, conducting clinical research studies of head and neck infections. We studied ear, sinus, and tonsil infections, and the Otolaryngology Clinic had nearly served as my second home for many years. I especially liked to work with resident physicians and help them with their research projects. Some of the studies we did had prevented surgical removal of the tonsils and improved the understanding of many infections. Because of these collaborations, I had the benefit of immediate access to the staff whenever I had any medical problem.

I saw Dr. Morell a few days after my return home. He examined me thoroughly and even performed an endoscopic examination, a test that enables the examiner to look directly inside the throat using a flexible tube as an optical instrument. The instrument not only provides an image for visual inspection and photography, but also enables biopsies, and it can even be used effectively in some minimally invasive surgery. Endoscopic procedures are generally painless and, at worst, associated with mild discomfort. I was happy that Dr. Morell performed the endoscopic examination because it is the most thorough means of establishing a diagnosis.

The examination took about two minutes and confirmed his suspicion that I was again experiencing reflux, a condition for which I had been previously diagnosed and medicated. He changed the acid-reducing medication I was already taking, hoping that it would work better than the old one. I was happy to hear that he did not find any other abnormalities.

Feeling reassured by Dr. Morell's findings, I followed his recommendations and resumed my busy schedule just as before. I had many things to take care of in a short period of time, as I had been working as an Infectious Diseases Physician in the US Navy for nearly twenty-six years and was approaching my age of retirement at sixty-five. I had no time to waste, for my retirement was only four months away. I had many research projects, numerous reports, and manuscripts to complete and could not afford the time for personal medical problems. Furthermore, the research institute I was associated with was interested in keeping me after my retirement, so I needed to prepare a research proposal to secure funding for continuous support of my research.

The sore throat ameliorated over the following weeks on the new medication, but a strange new sensation emerged – as if a piece of food was stuck in the back of my throat. I tried to cough it out and rinse it and even used my fingers to probe the area, but it did not help. I ignored the bothersome feeling for quite some time because I was very busy and out of town working most of the time, and I simply did not have time to seek medical help. Eventually, though, when the feeling did not subside, I finally went to see my otolaryngologist, Dr. Morell, on a Friday afternoon, arriving in his clinic directly from the airport.

I rarely used the unwritten privilege I had to walk in and ask to be seen right away. But this time, I instinctively felt that what I had might be more serious than reflux. I was very grateful for the privilege that I had to be seen at a moment's notice and often wondered how much delay happens in diagnosis and treatment of serious medical problems in patients who do not have such an easy access to specialists.

Even though it was late in the day, Dr. Morell saw me right away and performed a very detailed examination. To my surprise and dismay, he this time observed a new finding in the back of my throat which had not been there four weeks earlier. Using an endoscope, he observed a small polyp-like growth about the size of a small corn kernel (eight millimeters). Using a small monitor, I was able to watch as he maneuvered the endoscope and explored the new findings. In spite of what he had found, Dr. Morell did not seem alarmed and managed to do a good job of not raising my concerns by explaining away the new findings as a possible reaction to a foreign body such as a piece of fruit that got stuck in my throat just above the vocal cords. The small growth was behind the valve that closes when we swallow (the epiglottis) – the valve that prevents us from inhaling food into our lungs. I was able to feel the small mass because the valve hit it whenever I swallowed.

Although I was reassured by Dr. Morell's explanation that what I had was not serious in nature, his explanation did not make complete sense to me at the time because I did not recall having anything stuck in my throat and could not completely understand how a foreign body could induce such a growth so rapidly. When the doctor left the room for a minute, I questioned the junior resident who also observed the growth, asking her if she had ever seen such a foreign body. Even though she said she had not, I accepted Dr. Morell's explanation. *Who was I to question the opinion of the department chief?* Although head and neck infections are one of my major research interests, I am not an expert in visualizing foreign bodies in the back of the throat. I also wanted to believe that this was something simple and not anything serious. The thought that it could be cancer did not even occur to me, especially since my surgeon reassured me that this was very unlikely in my case, considering I don't smoke or drink and am therefore at a low risk of developing throat cancer.

Besides, I was too busy to worry. My oldest daughter was getting married in two weeks, and I could not afford a serious medical problem. *There are so many arrangements to be made,* I rationalized to myself, *and maybe I really do just have some piece of food stuck in my throat. I do tend to eat too fast and might have neglected to chew my food well.*

My doctor told me not to worry and advised me to see him again in a month. The irritation did not go away and became even more bothersome, so I decided not to wait a month. I returned to the Otolaryngology Clinic a week later on a Friday afternoon. Even though it was the second day of Passover and a non-working holiday for me, I had an appointment that afternoon at the Eye Clinic at the hospital. Since I was already in the hospital clinics and becoming increasingly annoyed by a worsening strange sensation in my throat (which was probably aggravated by eating matzos), I decided to see my otolaryngologist again. As before, he did not turn me away and repeated his examination. Again, he observed the small mass that seemed to have grown a little larger over the span of a week. I was able to see it myself on the special monitor and agreed with his assessment that it had grown larger in just a week's time.

This time, the doctor was more aggressive, but he still managed to remain calm and not raise my concerns. He offered to take a small piece of the mass (a biopsy) and send it for pathological examination. He looked for a special new biopsy kit that had just arrived in the clinic – one he had not used before – and after finding it, he attempted to perform the biopsy. However, he ran into some difficulties and needed assistance. Unfortunately, it was after four p.m., and the clinic was already empty. All the nurses, technicians, and other physicians who did work that day had already left for the weekend. He immediately offered an alternative.

"I am going to perform a biopsy on Wednesday of next week," he said. "This will be under general anesthesia, and you could go home in the afternoon."

Dr. Morell assured me it was a very minor procedure, and he seemed very unconcerned and underplayed his suspicion that it might be more than just a benign mass.

Now, I faced a dilemma. My daughter's wedding was in just nine days on the following Sunday. My wife and I were scheduled to fly to the west coast on Thursday and meet all the other members of our family who would also arrive on that day. The only one who would not be present was our youngest daughter, who was spending the second semester of her junior year of college in Cape Town, South Africa. There was too much at stake. We had been working hard to prepare for the upcoming wedding. If something would go wrong with my anesthesia or "minor surgery," everything would be spoiled. I even thought about my late father, who died from a sudden heart attack just three weeks before my wedding and never experienced the happy occasion. We had wanted to postpone our wedding after his sudden death, but the Rabbi insisted that it should proceed as scheduled, albeit without any celebration or dinner, insisting that it was the Jewish tradition. After that heartbreaking incident, I had always hoped to live long enough to experience my children's weddings. So now, with this impending "minor surgery," all I could wonder was, *Should I risk it? Should I undergo a potentially risky procedure so close to the wedding?* I wanted to live long enough to see more grandchildren and escort my other children to the wedding canopy. All of those thoughts and weighing all the odds for and against postponing the procedure went through my mind in a matter of few minutes.

After much deliberation, I felt that the risks of anesthesia, the minor surgery, and any potential discomfort were worth taking. Dr. Morell assured me that I would be in good shape to take the trip just one day after the biopsy, so I agreed to undergo the excision biopsy in five days.

I called my wife to tell her about the findings and the need for the biopsy. I tried to remain calm and underplay the potential of a serious illness. I also still believed, or wanted to believe, that this was something benign. My doctor was also reassuring me that this was nothing serious and that he had never seen any cancer that looked like the polyp I had. It seemed I was rather successful in not raising my wife's concerns, something I have always been good at. Even when I was a child, my mother taught me to avoid alarming people with potential bad news, and this was reinforced by years of practicing medicine. My wife tried to dissuade me from undergoing the procedure a day prior to the long trip and just three days before the wedding. She was concerned that I would have pain and discomfort that would detract from my ability to enjoy the happy occasion. In retrospect, she was correct, because I did experience all of these and more. However, I was driven by a gut feeling that this mass shouldn't be taken lightly — that it should be removed as soon as possible. *Who knows?* I thought, *If it is indeed cancer, who can tell when it will spread to the rest of my body?* I thought that even a week might make a difference.

Chapter 2. The Diagnosis

I worked hard during the five days before the biopsy and even drove from Washington DC to New Jersey to deliver a lecture on Monday night. Keeping my work schedule and staying busy helped me deal with the obvious anxiety prior to the procedure. I tried not to worry too much about what was waiting for me.

Early Wednesday morning, I arrived at the hospital for the biopsy. I came in unescorted as I had always done in the past when I had a procedure that did not require hospitalization. After all, this was a "minor procedure," and there was no need to trouble anyone. I told my wife not to worry about taking me home because one of my coworkers would check me out of the hospital after the procedure. Going through the admission process and putting on the patient gown were not new for me, although, as for anyone in that situation, there is always a tinge of apprehension. For me, it was somewhat difficult facing the fact that here, I was no longer a physician, but just one of the patients. I had my pulse, blood pressure, and temperature taken and waited for about an hour before they were ready to take me to the operating room.

I walked into the familiar preparation room that I had recognized from previous surgeries. It was a large room with about a dozen patient gurneys separated by curtains. Most of the gurneys were occupied by patients waiting for their turns to be wheeled into the operating room. The middle-aged woman across the room from me was waiting for a gynecological surgery, and a young man on my right was in need of knee repair.

Just like any other patient, I felt tense and nervous when I arrived at the waiting area. *Am I going to wake up after the anesthesia?* I began to shiver a little and asked for a blanket. What made the process of waiting easier was the friendly and upbeat atmosphere in the room created by the smiling personnel. A nurse took my medical history and started an intravenous line. I did not tell her that I was a staff physician. From past experiences, I had learned that the nurses had less trouble starting the infusion when they did not know who I was, which I assumed was because they were more relaxed and less apprehensive that way.

A friendly anesthetist examined me and looked at my throat to gauge the ease of intubating me. I assured him that I had been put to sleep in the past without any difficulty. I asked him, though, to be careful not to break any of my teeth while inserting the laryngoscope into my throat. I was reminded of my own difficulties during my medical training when trying to intubate patients – how, on one occasion, I slightly chipped the front tooth of an unfortunate patient while attempting to place a tube in his larynx.

I was always apprehensive about being intubated and under general anesthesia for surgical procedures. Whenever I needed minor surgery in the past, I always elected to stay awake and undergo the procedure, receiving only local anesthesia. This meant that on some occasions I had to endure more discomfort and even pain when the anesthetic wore off. I had always asked the anesthetist to administer the minimal amount of the general calming medication so that I could follow the progress of the surgery and, if possible, even watch it on a monitoring screen in the operating room. In reality, I rarely remembered details of the procedures, even when the dose of the medication was minimal.

The main reason I disliked being completely put to sleep was that that I did not want to lose control of the situation and did not have complete trust in the anesthetists. This fear was partially based on my own experiences early in my training some forty years earlier, when I witnessed mistakes that took place in the operating room. On one occasion, the anesthetist kept leaving the operating room to manage another patient in a different room, and on a second instance, the anesthetist failed to adequately ventilate a sleeping patient because the ventilation tube was incorrectly placed. Although these errors took place a long time ago and in a different country, I could not help but carry a deep-rooted mistrust of this particular part of medical practice.

My surgeon, accompanied by a young resident physician, stopped by for a few seconds just to say hello, and I was promptly wheeled into the operating room. It was a chilly, shiny, clean room full of surgical equipment and masked, gowned personnel. I was transferred to the operating table and noted that I was shivering again, either because of the scanty hospital robe and the chill in the room, or maybe because of my own anxiety. It was comforting to be covered by a warm blanket. The nurse placed electrocardiogram strips on my chest and connected them to the machine, and I was able to hear my own heartbeat. My blood pressure was taken again, and this time, it was slightly higher. Apparently, I was getting tense. The anesthetist slowly injected an anesthetic into my infusion and placed an oxygen mask on my face. Within seconds, I fell into a deep sleep.

I woke up in the recovery room. A nurse was attending me and taking my blood pressure and other vital signs. I was still very sleepy and confused, but as time passed, I slowly became more awake and oriented. I do not entirely recall the earlier events that occurred in the recovery room, but I learned later that the procedure took longer than expected, and about three hours had passed. As the anesthetic wore off, I started to feel intense pain in my throat and also felt nauseated. After an additional hour, I became more stable and was taken to the observation unit where I was to stay until I was released to go home.

However, even after hours passed, my nausea and pain did not subside sufficiently for me to be sent home. Consequently, my co-worker who came later in the afternoon could not take me home. He kept me company for a while, but I decided not to ask him to wait until I felt better and assured him that my wife would come later and take me home. My recovery was taking longer than I had experienced in the past. I called my wife, and she came to get me later in the evening after I felt better.

Fortunately, I had already packed up my bag in preparation for our upcoming trip to Los Angeles the next day. I was uncomfortable and coughed a lot but remained determined to tough it out and leave on time. This was one of the most joyful occasions in my life, and I was not going to allow a "minor procedure" to interfere with the event. Our schedule and itinerary were all calculated and tightly coordinated with the other members of the family, and there was no time for medical problems on that busy agenda.

My busy schedule distracted me from dwelling on the possibility that the biopsy might reveal something significant. A throbbing throat pain and cough kept me up at night, and I had some difficulty in swallowing. These were annoying reminders that I still did not know what the biopsy might reveal. I tried to remain optimistic, reminding myself, *Did not the surgeon assure you that what he saw does not look like cancer? Now, calm down.*

The next few days were truly happy and joyful. I felt fortunate to walk down the aisle with my daughter, co-signed the traditional wedding contract, and wished my blessing to her and her husband — all privileges my own father had missed. The thought occurred to me that even if I had a terminal illness, at least I was able to experience the wedding of my daughter. There were so many events, special meals, and ceremonies that I was completely consumed and almost forgot about the sword that still hung over my head. But occasionally, it did cross my mind. *What will the biopsy show? Oh, how I wish this "thing" did not exist.*

While waiting in the long security line at Los Angeles airport for my flight back on Monday morning, I called my surgeon to find out the results of the biopsy. The party was over, and I had to return to the realities of life. I was fortunate to have his direct number and was able to reach him right away. He told me that the results were not yet available and promised to contact the pathology laboratory to obtain them. He said this in his usual optimistic and cheerful voice, which kept me hopeful. However, I was annoyed at the continuous uncertainty. I wished he would have said, "It was just a benign lesion, nothing serious," but he didn't. I explained to him that I was about to board a plane for a five-hour flight and that I would arrive in Washington DC after he left his office. I asked him to leave me a message with the results on my answering machine. He promised to do that, and I boarded the plane for the flight.

During the flight (which seemed longer than usual), I tried not to think about the message that was waiting for me. I turned my cell phone on as soon as the plane landed and was rolling to the arrival gate. There was a single message waiting for me. I knew in my heart what it was about. My hands were shaking when I called to retrieve the message – a life or death verdict which would determine my future. I was hoping to hear a reassuring message that all was well. Through the noise and the stewardess's announcements on the plane's loudspeaker, I was able to hear my surgeon, and the news was not good or bad – rather, no news at all beyond a discouraging request for me to come to his office first thing in the morning to discuss the biopsy results.

I knew right away that this meant bad news. If the biopsy had not shown anything serious, he would have told me what the diagnosis was. I had skin biopsies taken before, and the dermatologists always left me a message with the benign findings. This was different; I could feel its ominous meaning. Doctors do not leave bad news on the phone. As soon as I deplaned, I listened to the message again, but I could not discern anything more. It was six in the evening, and the thought of waiting at least fourteen more hours seemed too difficult and wrenching. I wanted to know right then and there. I did not have Dr. Morell's cell phone or home number. I tried to get his home phone number from the phone book and telephone operator. I found three different telephone numbers which could be his, but none had the complete spelling of the first name. In my desperation, I even tried these three numbers, to no avail; no one answered my calls.

Fortunately, I was able to get the phone number of the otolaryngology resident on call for the hospital. I talked to him briefly, explaining my predicament, and asked him to contact my surgeon and ask him to call me with the biopsy results. Waiting in the airport for Dr. Morell's return call was unnerving. The resident called me back about twenty minutes later to inform me that my surgeon was in a meeting and could not call me back but asked me to come to his office in the morning.

I finally reconciled with the idea that I would have to live with the uncertainty overnight and that I should try to calm my growing anxiety. I was also determined to spare the potential bad news from my wife, who had returned to Washington on an earlier flight that day – at least until I learned more. In retrospect, I understand now why my surgeon could not have left me a telephone message, for this would have constituted an unethical and dangerous practice. In hindsight, I am also grateful that he did not spoil my ability to enjoy my daughter's wedding, as he had probably learned about the preliminary results much earlier. I wished, however, that I could have been spared the anxious hours that followed until I learned the truth.

Keeping the uncertainty and potential bad news from my wife was difficult. I did my best to hide my anxiety and worry, and it seemed to work well. I could not think about anything else, and my mind was racing and analyzing all potential interpretations of the message, its meaning, and its implications. The mundane tasks of unpacking and reading the mail occupied me, and I excused my silence as being tired after such a busy and eventful weekend.

Falling asleep was made more difficult by jetlag, but when morning came, I rushed to my surgeon's office. Dr. Morell had to go to the operating room that morning, and his secretary did not know when he would return. "He has a single case this morning and will come back as soon as he finishes in the operating room," she assured me.

My anxiety was so high that I could not wait any longer. I needed to know, and I decided to find out the results myself. I had visited the pathology laboratories many times before to inquire about my patients' results, but it felt very different this time. I passed through the long corridors that had the smell of formalin and other chemicals – halls I had wandered many times before, never feeling quite this vulnerable. I knew that dead patients were stored behind some of the closed doors and in the refrigeration chambers, and I was afraid that I would end up in one of those eerie places sometime in the not-so-distant future.

I tried to conceal my anxiety and approached the secretary in a professional, calm manner. "I need to see the results of the biopsy of a patient," I said. I was afraid that they would not let me see or hear the results if they knew I was inquiring about my own. The secretary was fooled by my subtle trickery, and I was allowed to see the pathology log book. Going down the list of samples from the day of the biopsy was like searching for my name on a death row roster. Following my name, the pathology log book read in no uncertain terms: "mildly differentiated squamous cell carcinoma."

I could not believe my eyes. *Is this possible? Can it be a mistake?* In spite of my mind's hopeful questions, I knew it was not a mistake – right here in front of me in black and white, my own death sentence. Suddenly, in that very instant, my whole world changed. I saw in front of me the unavoidable end. Strangely enough, I had always had a sense of invulnerability. I had been exposed to several life-threatening situations in the past and had always survived. I had never been deterred from taking physical risks, especially as a young man. In my twenties, I had been injured several times in motorcycle accidents, had been able to avoid hitting deer and other potential serious car accidents by quick reactions, and had participated as a medical corps physician in two wars when I lived in Israel, wounded in one of them. Yet, I had survived. I always felt that I had a lucky star. *Has my luck finally run out?* I wondered now, helplessly.

I had to accept for the first time that I am not invincible and that life has an end. I knew those things before, but I always trusted my body to stay healthy and avoid serious illness. I faced life-threatening situations when I participated as a medical officer at the ages of twenty-five and thirty-two in two wars the Six Days and Yom Kippur Wars. At those times, I felt I was simply not ready yet to die – I had not yet experienced life to its fullest, and there was so much more I wanted to do in life. During the Yom Kippur War, I was already the father of two young children and did not want to abandon them by succumbing to death. However, as I grew older, I slowly accepted the inevitability of illness and my ultimate mortality but hoped that they would occur in the distant future. I also felt that should death become inevitable, I could look back on my life and feel that I had done and experienced much of what I set out to do. Furthermore, unlike my father who died when my sister was only thirteen years old, all my children were adults, and all but one had finished their education and were almost completely independent.

My health until that moment had been generally good, and despite my age, I was in very good shape. I always seemed to recover or cope well with medical problems, and although I had several illnesses, they all turned out to be not so serious. But this? This was different. This was "mildly differentiated squamous cell carcinoma." At that minute, I thought, *This is it. This time, there is no chance that my illness will just go away.* My trust in my body to stay healthy and fit was lost.

On principle, I also had great difficulty dealing with the cancer diagnosis. I believed (wrongly, of course) that cancer was a lost cause, and once you have it, there is no way out. Even though I was interested in the research aspects of cancer, I had elected not to specialize in oncology. I was discontented with the futility of caring for patients suffering from cancer and chose instead to become a pediatrician and specialize in infectious diseases. Cancer is rarer in children, and most infectious diseases (especially in children) are curable. I had an inner prejudice about patients with cancer, feeling that they had an incurable illness and were bound to die – and soon. Oncology seemed like a doomed effort. During my years in medical school, I noticed that I was protecting myself from getting emotionally too close to patients with cancer so as not to feel pain when they passed away. In retrospect, forty years later, I realize these assertions are incorrect, because medicine has progressed so much since then. However, my previous superstitions were deeply imbedded in my mind and emerged at that minute when I read those haunting words: *Mildly differentiated squamous cell carcinoma.*

The only consolation I felt at that time was that I would be able to know ahead of time the cause of my death. In a strange way, I was expecting to die in a similar manner to my father, who died when he turned fifty-nine from a sudden heart attack. When I had my fifty-ninth birthday, I felt lucky that I had been able to pass that milestone. Unlike my father, I was more conscientious about my health, and I did not smoke like he insisted on doing. I also did not consume any alcoholic beverages. I felt that I might be more fortunate than my father who had died suddenly because I would have the opportunity to say goodbye to my family and friends. I had always felt that I had been granted an extension of my life when I survived my injuries from the Yom Kippur War. In that war, I was wounded in my leg by shrapnel, sustained an injury to my left eye, and fractured my orbit from the impact of an explosion which thrust me to the ground. I kept working and caring for other wounded soldiers for twenty more hours until I was evacuated to a hospital. I was lucky to have lived for many more years and more fortunate than some of my friends and many soldiers who had died during that war. I always felt I had been blessed with an extension of my life from the moment of my war injury and that all the years that followed were a bonus I was fortunate to have. All of these thoughts flooded my mind as I read the pathology report.

I asserted my stamina and behaved as if I were dealing with the results of someone else's biopsy and asked the secretary to direct me to the office of the pathologist who analyzed the biopsy. I was still in disbelief and, on some level, still hoping to hear from the pathologist that it was all a huge mistake. I also did not completely believe the results and wanted to look at the specimens with my own eyes. I needed a confirmation that this was true.

I was directed to the pathologist's office. It was a very strange situation for me. I have often visited the pathology laboratory to view my patient's pathological specimens. I believed in what I was taught during my medical training: there is no substitute to directly observing. This time, I was not asking to directly observe a patient's pathological slide, but my own.

I knocked on the door of the pathologist's office and walked in. It was a neatly set room with a large table at the center. A large microscope was situated in the middle of the table, and numerous specimen slides were scattered around it. The room had a strange odor of preservatives that made me slightly dizzy. The pathologist, a middle-aged woman, looked very professional and organized. "I am Dr. Brook from the Infectious Diseases Department, and I have just learned that the biopsy taken from my throat five days ago was found positive for cancer. Would you be able to review the specimen with me?" I asked. She did not flinch or show any emotion and willingly and politely agreed. We studied the pathological slides under the microscope together, and she explained the unique morphology of the cancer cells and how the diagnosis was made. Even though this was me and my life that we were talking about and I was looking at my potential killer, I amazingly was able to maintain my composure and act as if I was looking and discussing the results of a patient we both felt distant from – some stranger. However, it became clearer to me that there was no way out this time. This was truly a malignant tumor. I saw it with my own eyes this time.

Even though I had often studied pathological specimens of infectious processes, I had rarely observed cancer specimens since medical school. I recollected those as I viewed mine. This looked very familiar to me as I remembered the features of squamous cell carcinoma. Pathology was one of my favorite subjects in medical school, yet I always felt that I would never be affected by cancer. Nevertheless, it found me somehow. As I looked down into the slides and observed the cancer cells, I felt like I was gazing straight into the eyes of my nemesis. *This is going to kill me,* I thought.

The pathologist acted very professionally, and even though she had no comforting words, she eventually softened up and expressed her sorrow as being the one who had to deliver the bad news. I questioned her as to whether the whole tumor had been removed, and she assured me that it seemed to have been totally taken out. But she also cautioned me that even though the specimen she studied was surrounded by normal tissue, that layer was very thin. This meant that there was still a chance that the entire tumor had not been removed. I stoically took it all in and tried to express my feelings with a bit of dark humor. "At least I know what I will die of," I said to the pathologist.

With these parting words, I left her office carrying a copy of the pathology report and proceeded to my surgeon's office.

Chapter 3. Getting Started

I staggered back to the Otolaryngology Clinic, still shell shocked and bewildered. When I arrived there, my surgeon was already back in his office. His secretary, who had been my acquaintance for many years and had always helped me find him or another coworker, waved me in. It was a regular military doctor's office with his family pictures on his table and his framed medical degrees and professional and military awards hanging on the walls. There was a large model of a battleship that Dr. Morell must have served on proudly placed on a side table.

Dr. Morell was working on his computer when I knocked on the door. He immediately stopped what he was doing and gave me his full attention. I told him that I had already learned about the diagnosis, but he apparently had already learned about my visit to the Pathology Laboratory. The pathologist must have been alarmed by my last comment and called him. He explained the pathological findings to me and why he was able to remove only a minimal amount of tissue around the tumor. "It was difficult," he said, "to take out more tissue because the cancer was only a few millimeters away from the vertebral column. It is quite possible," he stressed, "that you are already cured. However, you need to receive radiation now, which is often the only treatment of this cancer. Even if some cancer cells were left, it will eradicate them."

Dr. Morell told me in calm and laid back tone how good my prognosis was because the cancer was detected at a very early stage, but he could not be specific about percentages of survival. Throughout the conversation, he was relaxed and seemed unconcerned and exhibited an upbeat spirit of optimism and experience, which helped me to better cope with the situation. He outlined my treatment plan, which would include only a course of irradiation to my neck, after which I would be followed in the Otolaryngology Clinic by the Tumor Board, monthly for the first year and at greater intervals later. They would be watching my recovery and making sure that I had no local recurrence or spread of the cancer to distant sites. That Board, a team of specialists in oncology, radiation oncology, endocrinology, dentistry, and otolaryngology, sees patients with cancer once a month. They would review my case and treatment plan later that week, after first reviewing the pathological and surgical reports, as well as the CT (computed tomography) and PET (positron emission tomography) scans. He had already ordered these scans to be done within the following twenty-four hours. The Board subsequently approved the plan of action he outlined to me.

Everything looked quite organized and in control, and this was reassuring. Without further delay, he told me that he had already talked about me to the radiation oncology specialists who were waiting to see me in their clinic. He personally escorted me downstairs to the clinic. As we were taking the elevator down into the basement, he told me that the pathologist had told him what I had said – that I now know what I would die of. His reassuring and surprising response was, "I am certain that this cancer will not kill you. You still need to take care of your health so that no other illness will cause it." It was good to hear that answer. It also reminded me that there were many other potential health hazards which I needed to watch for. Events in the future would prove how correct he was.

I realized that my surgeon's attitude was optimistic and positive because he tended to see the cup as half full and not half empty. In retrospect, I realized that his kind of attitude might have been a factor in his earlier lack of concern about the small lesion he had observed. This was probably why he was willing to wait a month and observe its progress rather than biopsy it right away, discounting the potential that it was malignant. On the other hand, I thought that he might have suspected cancer but decided not to raise my concerns and spare me the anxiety associated with sharing the potentials of that findings. I realized at that minute that I would always like to know the truth and my odds rather than having it concealed or painted in rosy colors. I asked him to promise me to always share the truth with me rather than hide it and protect me from it. He promised he would. He kept his promise and his door open for me in the ensuing months, just as he had done in the past, and he always found time to quell my anxieties and worries, examining me when needed without any delay.

The Radiation Oncology Clinic was situated at the basement of the hospital, probably because it contained heavy radiation emitting and monitoring equipment and thus requiring thick lead walls to protect the staff. Two radiation oncologists were waiting for us when we arrived at their clinic, an attending physician and a senior resident. They were friendly and smiling when they told me, "We were expecting you, Dr. Brook."

The senior resident reminded me by his looks of a good friend from medical school who now headed the Department of Oncology at a major medical center in Israel. They both had red hair, and similar facial features and mannerisms. I immediately felt a liking and connection to that resident who was to manage my case. *It is strange,* I thought, *how an irrational familiarity with superficial features sets my attitude and opinion of individuals.*

I was impressed and reassured by the radiation oncologists' self-confidence, knowledge, expertise and concern for my recovery. They outlined the treatment plan they had set for me, which included a series of thirty radiation sessions that would be given each week day for six consecutive weeks. They explained that they had new equipment and techniques that target the area of the tumor and spare the surrounding areas from excessive radiation. It was called "intensity modulated radiation therapy." I was wondering why they skipped the weekend days if the goal was to deliver a certain radiation dose to effectively kill the tumor. They assured me that it was okay to irradiate for only five days a week. I skeptically thought that this was just an excuse to close the facility over the weekend. I wanted to be treated every day so that the cancer would be eradicated as soon as possible. However, as I started to receive radiation and the side effects accumulated, I began to look forward to those two days of rest where some of those adverse affects ameliorated.

They outlined the side effects I would experience as a consequence of the radiation, including immediate and long-term. The almost immediate ones were change in taste, inflammation of the mouth mucosa with potential secondary yeast infection, skin irritation and hair loss at the area of irradiation, and tiredness. The long-term ones were thyroid hormone deficiency, scarring of the deeper neck tissues and muscles that would induce neck stiffness, damage to my nerves in the spinal cord and to the bones and roots of my teeth in the lower jaw, and the potential of development of malignancy. Although I was hearing about these complications, I was too overwhelmed and unable to appreciate their real meaning and severity. Only when I developed them did I truly understand their impact. Furthermore, at that time all of these seemed minuscule risks when compared to the task at hand – ridding me of the remaining cancer.

When I asked, "What are my chances for survival?" they gave varying estimates.

"Unfortunately," they explained, "most patients included in the published studies were diagnosed late, after the tumor had already reached a substantial size and had spread systemically. The later the diagnosis is made, the dimmer the outcome. The five years survival in advanced cases was dismal, only about 20 percent. However," they assured me, "your cancer was discovered at a very early stage, and those statistics may not apply to you. You have the best survival chance for patients with this type of malignancy. In those where the tumor is diagnosed and treated early, the chance of survival is much better and may reach 80 percent. "However," they stressed, "please understand that this is an unpredictable and difficult to treat type of cancer and has a relative high mortality rate. It does not respond well to chemotherapy, and very little improvement has occurred in the past three decades in both medical and surgical treatment. Please remember" they told me, "this kind of tumor generally spreads first to the local lymph glands, where it can stay checked for a while and only later spreads systemically – mostly to the lungs and liver. There is a chance of aborting the spread by early removal and treatment. On the other hand, there is always the possibility that the 'ginny has already got out of the box' and the cancer had spread. Unfortunately, there is no certain way to exclude that possibility, as even the most currently available sophisticated tests can not detect a very early spread."

I wanted to start receiving radiation therapy right away. I was afraid that any delay would allow the cancer to re-grow and spread. My surgeon's assertion that he "might" have removed all of it was not reassuring enough for me. My wife and I were planning to travel to South Africa the following week for two weeks. This trip was both professional and personal. I was invited to give a series of lectures in the major cities, and that would have also provided us an opportunity to visit our daughter, who was studying there, and a chance to tour the country and see some of the animal nature reserves. We had been planning that trip for months. I asked the radiation oncologists if a delay in starting the radiation treatment was possible, and they assured me that it would not pose a problem. However, that would mean that treatment would be delayed by three weeks. After I briefly considered the matter, I decided to cancel the trip and start treatment without any delay. No trip is worth giving up the chance of survival. I was disappointed that my treatment was only going to start a week later, as they needed that time to plan and calculate the doses and prepare a "mask" that fits my face and allows them to deliver an accurate dose of radiation.

I realized at that time that I had not yet shared the news with my wife and children, and it occurred to me that they should also be informed about what was going to happen. The radiation oncologists agreed to discuss my diagnosis and treatment with my children who were all residing in other cities. It was the reality of living in such a large country, as compared to life in small Israel where all family members typically live close to each other. After listening to the logic and potential prospects of success of the planned treatment, I wanted to share this with my family and alleviate their expected concerns and fears once I broke the news to them.

I left the Radiation Oncology Clinic in a better mood than I had before, feeling that I was in the good hands of a team of doctors who had my best interests in mind and knew how to handle it. However, there was still so much uncertainty about the future – about what kind I would have, and even how long it would be.

After leaving the clinic I broke the news to the Commanding Officer of the research institute where I worked and the head of my department. It was easier for me to do that than to inform my family. I also knew that it was my duty being in the military to let them know about my medical condition. The Commanding Officer is the officer everyone in the institute is under, and he or she has to be informed about any major issue pertaining to his personnel. Both were very supportive and understanding and promised to support me in any possible way. Ironically, that research institute is dedicated to studying the adverse effects of nuclear radiation – a topic I had researched for the past twenty-four years. I worked so hard to save people from the adverse effects of radiation, and now I was going to experience many of those untoward side effects myself.

The CT scan was completed that afternoon, and the PET scan was done the next day. These were sensitive tests that could detect cancer growth in the body. The CT is made of multiple X-rays that scan an area and can visualize abnormal growth, and the PET scan can observe a local increase in the consumption of sugar, which can indicate the presence of malignancy. However, neither test can detect lesions smaller than two centimeters, definitely unable to sense the presence of early cancer. Even though both tests were negative, I knew this did not mean I was necessarily tumor-free.

The next task I faced was the hardest. I had to tell everything to my wife. I decided to keep it from her for another night. I knew that our world would be entirely different afterwards, and I wanted to spare her a night of agony and give her another evening of normality. It was not easy to keep it from her, especially because she was still planning the upcoming trip overseas. I tried to distract her from spending too much time on planning the trip. She kept reading about the places we were going to visit and talking to me about the hotels where we were to stay. I knew that it was all futile and that we were not going to take the trip. I kept wondered how to best break the news to her.

We had a brush with cancer a year earlier when a suspicious mammogram brought up the possibility of breast cancer in my wife. It was a very traumatic and emotionally draining experience for me. I felt that my whole world was falling apart until a biopsy showed no cancer. I had not yet completely recovered emotionally from that traumatic experience, and now we were going to be thrust into one where I was the sick one. And this time, it was not just a cancer *scare*, but a *reality*. How would my wife cope with it?

I was also flooded by thoughts of despair, helplessness, and depression knowing I now had to deal with cancer. However, I had so many things to do, and I felt an inner sense of hope that I could do something proactive that would eradicate the rest of the cancer. Knowing this helped me push aside the negative thoughts. These returned, however, to haunt me again and again.

Early the next morning, I decided to tell my wife what had happened. I thought the morning would be a better time to deal with bad news than the evening. The morning was better time I thought because she was not tired and could reason with clarity and have the whole day to deal with the news, hopefully resolving the issues by nightfall so as not to miss a night's sleep. Even though I knew I had to finally deliver the bad news, I was not sure when, exactly, I should do it. I kept postponing it again and again during the morning. I wanted her to eat first and get dressed, but time was running out. She was making her final preparation to leave the house for work and taking out a few items from the walk-in closet when I approached her.

The support, information, and treatment plan I obtained on the previous day made me stronger and more ready to support her and provide her with an optimistic outlook and plan of action. I kept all my fears and worries about the uncertainties to myself. I delivered the bad news as tactfully as I could. I started by saying "I am afraid that we may not be able to travel to South Africa because of a new medical problem I had developed." I than proceeded to explain why. She was stunned and speechless. She opened her mouth in disbelief and could not utter a word for almost twenty seconds. I proceeded immediately to tell her that I may already be cured, but just to be sure that there is no cancer left, I was going to receive radiation treatments. I also informed her that my CT scan was negative and that to hear more details, we would be meeting the radiation oncologists that afternoon. It seemed to have worked, and although my wife was initially shaken, she seemed to absorb the news and started processing and adjusting to the new reality we were facing.

We met the radiation oncologists later on that day. They repeated the reassuring well-structured explanations they gave me on the previous day. My confidence in them was also comforting to my wife, and we left the clinic feeling we had a plan of action that may lead to recovery.

The next task was to inform our children. This was difficult, as we could not do it in person but had to do it by phone. We did it as delicately as possible, reassuring them of the good prognosis and outlining the treatment plan. They accepted the news with great concern. Fortunately, they all had full lives that kept them busy. We did not get in touch right away with my oldest daughter, who was overseas for her honeymoon, but waited for her return, for we did not want to spoil her happiness. What was very helpful was that our children had the opportunity to talk with the radiation oncologists, who provided them with detailed information and answered all their questions and concerns. I was very grateful to the radiation oncologists for providing their services to all my family members and assisting us in coping with these uncharted waters.

Informing our daughter in South Africa was more difficult, especially as we were about to visit her. It was hard to ascertain her reaction because she was so far away. She cried when she heard the news. After we succeeded in calming her down a little, she had many questions and was very upset and distraught. It took some time to explain to her the situation and try to leave her less distressed. We had, of course, to tell her that we were not going to visit her, which was also very disappointing to her.

At that time, I had to decide if I would like to share my diagnosis and condition with other family members, friends, neighbors, and colleagues. I decided to keep it private and share it only with my wife and children and those colleagues who needed to know. I asked my wife and children to respect my choice. Some of them tried to convince me to change my mind because silence imposes an additional burden upon them, where they cannot share their anxieties and worries with others. Still, though, they all promised to comply with my request, even though some found it hard. Our daughter, who was in South Africa at that time and had no family support, asked my permission to confide with some close friends, to which I agreed. I was trying to understand myself why I wanted it that way and came out with several reasons. One was that I did not want to show my vulnerability and weakness and be pitied by others. I felt that my illness was my own private issue and that it was my prerogative to determine whom I want to share it with.

The other reason I wanted to keep it private was because I did not want to be stigmatized and discriminated against. I knew that sick people – especially those with potentially terminal illness – are less able to be competitive in society and are intentionally or unintentionally discriminated against. I experienced the painful stigmatization some time later when a close relative expressed fear that that I will "infect" her infant with cancer if I share my spoon with her.

I was also afraid that otherwise compassionate friends and acquaintances might distance themselves from me to protect themselves from the inevitable – knowing that they may lose me to my affliction with a malignant cancer. I based this fear on my own prejudices and my own reactions to other sick individuals, although whenever I had to face terminal illness in friends I never acted that way. When two of my close friends were diagnosed with cancer, I kept visiting and supporting them all the way. Still, I just felt that I could better cope with my situation if I kept it private until I was strong enough to reveal it.

I had about a week before the radiation treatment started. I did not change my schedule and worked as planned. I even traveled out of town to deliver two lectures. I did, however, cancel all other activities for the upcoming six weeks, including the trip to South Africa. I felt bad about doing that, especially at the last minute, because I prided myself as a professional who always fulfilled his commitments and obligations. Bad weather or illnesses were rarely a cause for cancellation. This time, though, it was all different.

We canceled all of our reservations in South Africa and, to our surprise, the hotel managers in all these places returned our deposits when they understood why we had to cancel at the last minute. It was a gesture that warmed my heart and made me feel that people we have never met really do care.

During the week preceding the radiation treatment, I had a series of appointments in various clinics where my medical and dental conditions were checked to form a baseline prior to treatment. These checkups included a dentist, a dental hygienist, and a dietician. When I broke the news to my internist, he did not utter a word until he gave me a big supportive hug. It felt so good to know that he deeply cared for me beyond our professional realm. I had never been hugged by a medical caregiver or given a hug to a patient. His embrace moved me and made me feel that I was surrounded by caregivers who truly appreciated my pain and distress and shared in my personal tragedy. I also contacted the social worker I had seen several years ago. I felt I needed to talk to her with and without my wife so that we could better cope with this life-shaking event and its repercussions. From my past experience with her, I knew that her assistance would be invaluable. This was a very wise decision, because we needed and benefited from her caring, compassionate, and wise advice in the following months and years. She helped us cope with the ups and downs and the fears and anxieties that followed; she was a constant source of help and support. With her assistance, I actually became more resilient.

I went to the Radiation Oncology Clinic during that week to have a special fenestrated mask prepared that snugly fit my face. That mask, specially molded for me, was to be worn by me every time I received radiation. It prevented me from moving my head and neck during the radiation session and insured the precise delivery of the radiation dose to the tumor site. It was prepared by softening the mask in hot water, placing it on my face for a few minutes while it was cooling off, and leaving it on my face until it solidified. It resembled the fencing mask I used to wear when I practiced that sport during my student days. This mask bore my name and was there waiting for me each time I went in for radiation. They told me when they prepared the mask that I could take it with me at the end of therapy as a souvenir; however, when I finally finished the long and grueling treatment, I declined the offer. I did not want to possess anything that would remind me of that experience.

After completing the mask, the technicians etched a small black point in the middle of my chest. This was done to enable them to direct the radiation beam in an exact fashion. I was tattooed for life – literally.

A few months later, I checked into an airport hotel in Charlotte, North Carolina, on a rainy night. After taking a few steps into the hotel's lobby, I slipped and fell on the floor. The guests' umbrellas had dripped onto it, making it a slippery sheen. I approached the front desk to complain about my injury and to request they promptly dry the floor to avoid further accidents, and the hotel manger came to talk to me. He was an elderly man, skinny and tall. He apologized and suggested that I file a form with the hotel insurance company for my injured hand. After talking to him for a few minutes, I learned that he had experienced a type of malignancy similar to mine and had also been treated with radiation. I asked him if he had also received a tattoo on his chest. He untied his tie and unbuttoned his shirt and showed me the same mark. I felt immediate camaraderie with him, realizing that there must be many survivors like him bearing a similar "mark of Cain" as a souvenir. After all, we both shared the same turbulence and experiences. I refrained from following up on my formal complaint or filling the insurance forms simply because I did not want to get a fellow survivor in any trouble. He had been through enough already, as I knew firsthand all too well.

Chapter 4. Getting Irradiation

The beginning day of the radiation series finally came, and I arrived at the clinic early in the morning. I used the Metro train instead of driving my car, as I was not sure how I would feel afterwards. I avoided driving throughout the course of my radiation treatment, and for weeks later, because I felt very insecure when I tried to drive after treatment, constantly fearing I would have an accident. The clinic was located in the hospital basement, staffed by very efficient and friendly personnel. When I walked in and sat waiting for my turn, I noticed there were a few other patients waiting with me. They all obviously had cancer and shared similar treatment regimens. Some looked very healthy and fit, but most looked ill and worn out – as if they had endured much pain and suffering.

Am I going to look like that in a few weeks? I wondered. After a time, I began to recognize some of the frequent visitors, but we never did strike up conversations beyond greeting each other. Everyone kept their story to themselves. This was a group of strangers, united only by a common personal tragedy and a similar hope to benefit from radiotherapy. I often wondered what kind of cancer each of them had and how successful their treatment would be. A few were relatively young, and I felt especially sorry for them, as they were being afflicted with cancer in the prime of their lives. Many were elderly gentlemen, probably military retirees, considering that this was a military institution. I wondered what they had done in their lifetimes and what military ranks they had held. *Have they been in wars, exposed to the*

31

tragedy of losing friends in combat? Have they faced the threat of death dur-ing war like I did? Did these experiences make them more resilient? Did they smoke and drink during their long and lonely deployments and is that why they now have cancer? I would have liked to know their stories.

Some were women, of course, and most of them covered their hair to conceal the secondary hair loss from chemotherapy. I assumed that many of these women were suffering from breast cancer.

It was a very strange feeling to sit in the waiting room among fellow cancer victims and be one of them. I remembered that several years ago when I had mild anemia and had been examined at the com-bined Hematology/Oncology Clinic, I felt very uneasy to be there. The waiting room there was more comfortable and had more ameni-ties than in other clinics in the hospital, and the medical personnel were very compassionate and friendly. I thought then that this was probably because everyone wanted to make the life of those unfor-tunate individuals happier, as they may not live very long. Most of the patients at that clinic had cancer and looked quite ill. I felt very sorry for them, knowing that they were struggling for their lives, but I had the comfort of knowing that I was not one of them. Whenever I was among those cancer patients, I wanted to wear some kind of tag on my shirt that said, "No, I'm not dying of cancer like everyone else in here" – something to show that I was not one of those destitute patients. I had been very biased and irrational in my thoughts and beliefs about cancer back then, stigmatizing those with it as hopeless cases. But now, I no longer felt that way. *Now I'm one of them – a cancer patient myself, but I am going to get better,* I thought.

Even though I had become one of *those* patients, I did not feel helpless. I wanted to conquer the disease, believing in the power of the invisible radiation rays to clean up the sites the surgeon's knife could not or did not reach. Walking into the clinic that morning felt good, as if I was being proactive and was finally fighting back by 'cleaning my house'. I was beginning a struggle, of course, a struggle that might root out the remaining cancer cells that might still be lurking in my body.

After changing into a hospital gown, I was lead by the technicians to the room where the radiation was to be delivered. Several monitoring screens were present outside the room, which enabled the staff to observe and control the equipment inside the room. There were many yellow and red warning signs that alerted everyone about the danger of radiation exposure. The thick bank-style safety metal door was to be closed tightly during my treatment, but the technician assured me that I would be constantly watched and could call for help at any time by ringing a bell. There was a small operating room-style table in the center of the room, and hovering over it was a huge radiation emitting machine, similar to an X-ray. Waiting for me on the wall and bearing my name was my face mask.

I was strapped to the table, and the mask was tightly fitted on my face, and then the mask itself was tightly fixed to the table. I could see and breathe through it, but it was hard to get used to the tight fit. The radiation was to be delivered over a period of about twenty-five minutes, and I was to stay still and not move the upper part of my body. Since I was still coughing a lot, I was afraid that it would be difficult for me to suppress a cough during the procedure. When I asked "What should I do if I have to cough?" the technicians assured me that they would promptly stop the radiation and come in to release me. I was skeptical that they would be able to respond in a timely manner and hoped that I would never need to do that. Fortunately, even though it was not easy at times to control my urge to cough, I never had the treatment interrupted.

Before starting the radiation session, the technicians completed a series of X-rays to make sure that my position in relation to the radiation source was optimal. I noted that they did not place any shield over any radiation sensitive sites on my body such as my liver, spleen, or genitalia. *This is odd,* I thought, *I have always taken great care to protect these parts whenever I've had diagnostic X-rays.* Whenever I had researched radiation effects during the past twenty-four years, I was extremely careful to avoid unnecessary exposure. I always wore a small, credit card-sized radiation monitoring device that would have alerted me about any untoward exposure. But now I realized that I was no longer a person that should be protected from radiation.

The floodgates for radiation had been lifted, and precautions that had been engrained in me by my very profession did not apply to me any longer. I was to receive so much radiation in the near future that protecting me from exposure to several X-rays would not make a significant difference. Indeed, those X-rays became routine in most of the following sessions, as the accurate delivery of the radiation depended on them. I no longer had to be protected from developing cancer anyway, because I had it already. I became a "person of a lesser class." Now, I was the irradiated one – like the laboratory mice I had experimented on during my research. I was unable to voice my concerns, as the mask I wore prevented me from speaking, but I did not voice them even when the mask was off. I just accepted my new reality of being dispensable and stigmatized.

The technicians left the room, and the metal door was shut tightly. I was left alone in the room facing the enormous radiation emitting machine that was hovering over me. Soon, the machine started moving, producing robot-like sounds, and started rotating from my left to my right. It rested for a few minutes at eight fixed locations where it delivered its invisible deadly dose. I knew that I was getting exposed to huge amounts of radiation. I was worried about my unprotected eyes and brain, although the doctors had assured me that these organs could tolerate the radiation well. Even though the whole experience was unnerving and strange, I felt good that I was finally beginning to fight back in an effort to eradicate the cancer.

Over the weeks that followed, I got accustomed to the routine. It was, however, very uncomfortable, and I could not wait for each session to end so that I could be released from the tight mask and get up and leave. I began to calculate how many sessions I still had left before the ordeal would be over. Each time the radiation machine would complete a single delivery of its dose, I calculated how many more were left and what percentage of the total I had left to endure. I knew that I was getting closer and closer to the end after each dose.

Even though the treatments were difficult to bear, I was very eager to get treated. When the clinic was closed for an extra weekend day because of Memorial Day, I protested and inquired if it would be wise to stop the pounding of my cancer for three days in a row. Complaining did not help, because all the hospital clinics were closed over that holiday anyway. So, I had to wait and hope it would not make a difference.

When a computer problem forced the cancellation of the radiation therapies for five consecutive days, I was very upset. I insisted that they either get the problem fixed or send me to be treated at a different facility so that my treatment would not be interrupted any longer. I was determined to do my best to achieve a cure and not allow any technical problems to stand in the way. As an infectious diseases specialist, I knew that one could not stop antibiotic therapy over the weekend or even longer without serious consequences. This was not, perhaps, the case with cancer, but I sensed that my doctors did not know for certain what was best. After threatening to speak with the hospital Commanding Officer, I had my treatment continued after hours at the National Institutes of Health (NIH) until the problem with the computer was resolved. This was relatively easy, I understood later, because the equipment at NIH was identical. The senior radiation oncologist also had credentials at NIH, and he and the radiation technologist came with me and personally delivered the radiation sessions. I was the only patient that got treated in that fashion and wondered why others were not sent to other places as I had been. Unlike me, most of them probably did not push for it.

I started to feel the untoward effects of the radiation right away. Immediately after getting up and leaving the room, I experienced intense exhaustion and disorientation, which lasted a few hours. Fortunately, that occurred only during the first couple of weeks. However, I started to feel general fatigue and a lack of energy that increased over time. I changed from a person who had been very productive to one who could do very little. I spent many hours just dozing off.

Fortunately, the World Cup Soccer Tournament was taking place during that period, which allowed me to watch the games and rest.

As it so happened, soccer had played a major role in my childhood and even though I liked watching the game, I rarely had time for it anymore. Ironically, my incapacity freed me to return to my early interest. My father was a soccer player in the 1930's and a member of one of the best soccer teams in Austria, the Jewish team of Hakoach Vienna, and then in British Palestine, where he was a member of the Jewish National soccer team. My mother and I used to join him when his team traveled all over the country for soccer league games, and I spent many weekends with him watching his team play even after he had retired from the game. I was not as talented as my father when it came to playing mid-field, but I excelled as a goalkeeper and often played with my friends until I got more interested in studying. In spite of my illness, it was good to have this "forced respite" to enjoy a game I had long been detached from but enjoyed very much.

As time passed, the radiation's untoward effects started to intensify, affecting me in various ways. I experienced increasing pain and dryness in my throat, and gradual changes in taste made it difficult for me to eat. These worsened with time until they became unbearable at the end of the course of therapy. Almost everything tasted bad. The best I could expect was for the food to be bland and have no taste at all. As time elapsed, I developed an aversion to more and more foodstuffs. The intensifying pain and sore throat were a growing stumbling block, preventing me from eating or enjoying anything I could manage to ingest. Solid food was especially difficult to chew and swallow. I was warned that maintaining my weight was essential, for loss of weight might have serious deleterious effects. I was warned that if I stopped eating or drinking, I might need to have a feeding tube placed into my stomach through a hole in my abdominal skin. I could become dehydrated, which would mandate hospitalization to receive intravenous fluid. During my course of treatment, I observed several patients who were brought to the clinic in wheelchairs, connected to feeding tubes or intravenous fluid lines. This strengthened my resolve to do my best to take in what foods and beverages I could. I did not want the added burden of tubes and lines.

Even though I had little appetite, I forced myself to eat and constantly searched for food items that I had not yet developed an aversion to. I looked for high-calorie, small-volume foods – the kinds most dieters would hastily avoid. In the early weeks of treatment, I was able to eat soft food and soup, but after a while, I could not even consume those. I ended up surviving on water, watermelon, jello, ice cream, sour cream, and some yogurt. I no longer worried about gaining weight or consuming too much fat or cholesterol. All items of food, including my favorite ones, now tasted awful. At the end of the six weeks of treatment, I was almost at the point where I was unable to swallow anything. It was a constant struggle to keep my weight from declining. I had done a good job in preventing the need for tube feeding or hospitalized because I lost only seven pounds through those grueling six weeks and the slow recovery period.

My throat became extremely painful, beefy red, sensitive, and very inflamed, and my saliva production declined, causing me to have a very dry mouth. It took a few months for those symptoms to recede after I ended the radiation treatment. However, the saliva production never recovered completely, and my taste changed. To reduce the pain, I was prescribed a liquid mixture of topical anesthetics that provided only temporary relief. To decrease my pain after each treatment, I walked over to the ice cream store on the hospital grounds and ate a small scoop of vanilla ice cream, hoping to cool my throat after the radiation treatment and perhaps absorb some of the radiation energy.

Another gradually worsening side effect of the radiation was the burn-like effect on my skin. This included pain, redness, and inflammation of the skin around and below the neck. The topical creams I received alleviated some of the irritation. All the hair in these areas stopped growing. This was the only thing I did not mind, because I did not have to continue my daily shaving routine which I always disliked anyway. To my disappointment, a month after the radiation treatment ended, the hair starting growing back, and I had to resume shaving.

I had suffered from several side effects in the first two to three weeks of my treatment that included tiredness, headaches, and cloudiness of my perception. I realized after a while that my treating resident and attending physicians were becoming impatient and were sometimes irritated when I came to them for advice and support. One of them told me that I should not feel so tired so early in the course of treatment. He also told me that I should wait for my weekly examination to voice my questions and concerns.

I was surprised and upset by his seemingly callous attitude. I could not explain why I experienced symptoms so early, but I knew that medicine has no set rules and that people differ in their reaction and timing of side effects. I needed the doctors to be there for me. Everything was so new to me. I was used to being energetic and lucid, so I was concerned and worried about my symptoms and looked to them for advice on how to cope. I also needed reassurance that these were expected side effects and that they would go away afterwards. To my relief, those symptoms diminished in intensity in the remaining weeks. Where other patients generally feel worse over time, I somehow adjusted to the growing intensity of some of the side effects and surprisingly felt less tired and had fewer and fewer headaches. I was relieved that I did not have to bother the physicians and ask them for advice anymore. Fortunately, I found more receptive ears and got helpful advice from the clinic nurse.

The clinic had a very structured protocol of taking care of its patients. I was weighed, and had a complete physical examinations and discussion with the doctors on a regular weekly basis. Furthermore, the clinic nurse was always willing to respond to my questions, concerns, and any medical problem that arose. She was very compassionate and had a very optimistic approach, which was especially helpful and often came with practical solutions and advice that she learned from many years of experience.

The accumulation and worsening of the radiation side effects made it harder and harder for me to endure. I understood for the first time why some patients with terminal illnesses who have to endure such painful and debilitating modalities of treatment elect to forgo them.

It may be temping at the peak of side effects to quit and accept the inevitability of their situation and choose palliative treatment only. I thought about quitting several times. But in the end, I chose to hang in sometimes just because I was too tired, not able to think lucidly, and too exhausted to change my routine of coming every day to be irradiated. Despite the lose of energy and drive, I kept coming again and again to get my daily radiation treatments like a fatigued boxer who just wants to make it to the last round standing on his own two feet, no matter how bloodied and wobbly he is. I wondered why there was no better way to cure cancer than this almost century-old method – such a very crude and destructive one, damaging so many healthy body structures because it did not discriminate between cancer cells and normal ones. I wished that there were a better and easier way to treat cancer.

Strangely, all desperate and depressing thoughts that kept entering my mind lost their intensity as my fatigue and inability to concentrate intensified. Paradoxically, these negative side effects helped me push aside these troubling thoughts enough to go on with my treatment. I was simply too tired to will myself away from the very thing that was making me tired.

When I look back at those six weeks and the period of recovery that followed, it feels like a bad dream that faded away with time. I cannot recollect many of the details and events during that period, especially as my general exhaustion and fatigue worsened.

Early on in the course of my treatment, I experienced the joy and celebration of one of the patients when his radiation course was completed. He came for the last visit accompanied by his close relatives who brought a cake, candy, and soft drinks for the staff. At this stage, I did not understand why getting to the end of therapy was such a milestone and cause for celebration. However, I came to appreciate this at the end of my own treatment, although I did not wish to have a formal party. I knew that my struggle was not yet over, and I hoped there would be time and cause for partying later.

Chapter 5. Life After Irradiation

I was walking down the street back from the hospital after the last radiation session knowing that I was finally free from grueling six-week radiation ordeal. Even though I should have felt a great sense of exhilaration, I was too mentally numb and too physically exhausted to sense anything. Yes, I had made it to the finish line, but I still felt tired and consumed. I knew I still had to face a slow, long recovery. It was good, however, to experience the gradual return of my sense of well-being and lessening of exhaustion. My energy returned slowly, and I was able to resume greater amounts of physical activity. My general feel of malaise and inability to think and plan ahead slowly dissipated. These improvements correlated and were probably augmented by the subsiding of inflammation and the disappearance of the throbbing pain in my mouth and throat. The process was gradual and took two to six months, complete with ups and downs as other late appearing side effects emerged over time.

The lengthy recovery period was accompanied by the emergence of a series of newer side effects, many of which were lifelong. I was forewarned by the radiation oncologist to expect some of them, but I was unprepared and surprised by others they never told me about. When some of the late side effects of radiation started to appear, I became unsettled and unsure what new adverse effect would come next. My physicians avoided responding to my question, "What else can happen to me?" They told me about the major side effects (such as low thyroid gland function and neck stiffness), but I wish they would have been more open and honest with me about all the potential repercussions of the radiation treatment. If they would have provided me with more information, I would have been less concerned and apprehensive when these side effects actually emerged. I had the feeling that they avoided talking to me about all of the potential side effects because they were unable to predict with any certainty which ones I would likely experience and perhaps hoped that I would not have many.

The first new adverse effect that manifested itself about three months after the end of the radiation treatment was a sensation of electrical impulses that ran from my lower spine down into my legs whenever I bent my head down. I was very scared and concerned when I first noticed it. I was in Atlanta, Georgia, giving a series of lectures when I first felt these electrical shocks and, being unaware what they were, I was afraid that they represented a cancer invasion in my spinal cord. I felt them late at night and became terrified when I sensed them. Fortunately, they occurred on the last night of my three-day trip. I was able to send a detailed email message to my radiation oncologist explaining my symptoms before leaving for the airport.

Upon my return to Washington, I rushed to the hospital. I was prepared for the worst. The radiation oncologist welcomed me with a big smile and, without even listening to me, handed me a few pages. "Read them, and you will be relieved," he said. I glanced at the Internet printouts that discussed in detail the symptoms I had and ascribed them to what is medically called "L'hermitte's Sign," named after the doctor who first described them. Apparently, this complication can occur in about ten percent of patients who receive radiation to the neck or spine area.

He explained to me that radiation therapy can cause damage to the spinal nervous system because these structures were included in the radiation field. My tumor was a few millimeters away from the spine, which was why it was exposed to substantial amount of radiation. The condition is believed to be due to temporary demyelization of the posterior columns of the spinal cord. These nerves were not functioning well and misfired when stimulated by stretching. He assured me that no intervention was required, and the syndrome usually resolves spontaneously over a period of months to one year. I felt a great sense of relief after I heard this explanation. Suddenly, the fear of the unknown was lifted, and there was something concrete to hang on to. *Why did you not tell me about this before it happened?* I wanted to scream at him. *I could have been spared so much anxiety and distress!*

Although the condition worsened in the ensuing months, it did dissipate over time, but never disappeared completely. A neurologist that I consulted advised me that although the damage to the nerves is permanent, my brain learns to ignore the electrical shocks over time, and they become less noticeable.

The other permanent side effect was the emergence of low thyroid gland function (or hypothyroidism). The thyroid gland is an important endocrine gland in the neck, and mine was in the field of radiation and was expected to be permanently damaged. This gland produces the thyroid hormones, which are critical determinants of metabolic activity and affect the function of virtually every organ system. The symptoms were insidious in the beginning, and I attributed them initially to the lingering general tiredness after radiation, but they worsened with time. I developed extreme fatigue and weakness, depression, constipation, loss of breath on exertion, and cold intolerance.

My radiation oncologist advised me not to worry about hypothyroidism until four months after the end of radiation, but in my case they came sooner – about ten weeks later. I re-learned what I had already known from my years of study: there really are no set rules in medicine, and every individual is unique in their response to radiation. I brought the presence of these symptoms to the attention of my doctors and insisted that they measure my thyroid hormone blood levels. The deficiency in my thyroid activity was immediately diagnosed, and hormone replacement treatment was started. Unfortunately, it took a few months for the symptoms to disappear. This was partially due to the slow nature by which clinical improvement of hypothyroidism occurs and also because the exact dose of the hormone needed for replacement is individual and cannot be predicted.

My treatment was started with a low hormone dose, and a stable equilibrium had to be achieved, which took about six to eight weeks. The blood levels were determined, and the dose was adjusted accordingly when needed. This was a tedious process that took several months before the correct replacement dose was achieved. What complicates the situation even more after radiation is that the process of deterioration in the activity of the thyroid gland may take a few months, during which the required replacement dose increases. It took almost five months in my case for the correct daily dose to be determined.

I lacked energy to perform even simple tasks. I was tired and wanted to sleep all the time. I noticed that my thought process was very slow and restricted, I was forgetful, and I lacked interest in anything. I had no energy left to do any activity. I felt unmotivated to read or write, go the movies, bike, or even take short walks. I only did the essentials. My spirits were down, and I avoided leaving the house, walking around in a tired and sleepy funk. It was especially difficult over the weekend to excuse my behavior to my wife who worked all week and wanted to go places and do things together. I felt very guilty and apologetic when I was unwilling to join her. After I understood the cause of my tiredness, I did my best to explain to her that all of this was temporary and would go away and there was nothing that is permanently wrong with me. But I was afraid that this was not convincing enough. I looked normal, but was still a basket case.

To make matters worse, I had a creeping depression that made everything even harder. I was trying very hard to deal with the aftermath of being diagnosed with cancer, and the new physical disability made it much harder.

It was hard for me to feel the positive effects of the lifting the veil of symptoms of hypothyroidism that were so disruptive of my life. However, after a few months of patience and perseverance in taking the replacement thyroid hormone and having the dose adjusted to my needs, things felt slowly better, and I began gradually returning to my old self. I was feeling that I was slowly emerging from a nightmare back into real life – but a different kind of life, in the shadow of cancer. Once I regained my clarity of mind, I came to the realization for the first time of the full impact of what I would have to live with – the uncertainty of the future and what waits for me next. *Will the cancer return? When will it happen? How can I make long-term plans, or should I even try to? In case it does come back, what things should I do to conclude unfinished business?*

Neck stiffness was a constant and an annoying result of the exposure of my neck muscles to irradiation. It limited my range of neck motion, and I felt frozen in my position. I tried to break the freeze and regain more motion by exercising and was slowly able to achieve greater flexibility. However, I was warned by my doctors that this was going to be a constant challenge throughout my lifetime as the post-radiation muscle stiffness was never going to fully disappear.

I noticed that my vision was also affected. I needed two adjustments of my reading glasses and noticed cloudiness in my field of vision (a sign of cataract development) in the months that followed the radiation. I suspected that the exposure of my lens to radiation generated these changes.

Sixteen months following radiation, I developed high blood pressure that required medication. Although this might have been age-related, there was a strong possibility that this was the result of scarring of the blood pressure sensors that regulate the blood pressure in the carotid artery that runs through the neck, which was exposed to radiation. I inquired about the possible connection between radiation and the development of high blood pressure with my otolaryngologist, radiation oncologist, and internist, and they just shrugged their shoulders and admitted their ignorance in this topic. I decided to explore the issue myself and after spending just a few minutes on the Internet I found out that investigators at the NIH had described and studied several patients with this condition. I called the scientist who had performed that study and asked to be seen by him, but he told me that he no longer works on that topic. He also informed me that even if the high blood pressure is the result of the radiation, the treatment is the same. To my disappointment, when I informed my doctors about the study at NIH, most seemed skeptical. I thereafter accepted the reality of the situation and followed the recommendations of my internist, and with proper medications my blood pressure returned to normal. But unfortunately, the problem was not over.

Almost three years after I received the radiation, I experienced an unexpected and unexplained episode of fainting and started to suffer from dizziness. Tests by a cardiologist revealed that I had developed a tendency for low blood pressure when I stand up. He agreed with me that this newly developed blood pressure instability might have been the direct result of radiation of the neck. Unfortunately, he could not offer any solution for my problem except to lower my blood pressure medications and accept a higher blood pressure so that fainting would not happen again.

I was frustrated by the inability of any of my doctors, regardless of all their specialties, to help me, and I wondered if my problem was just too rare for them to recognize it. I decided to visit webwhispers. com, the wonderful support site for laryngectomy patients. I posted a question asking if anyone had also suffered from dizziness after radiation of their neck. Within six hours of placing the question, I received over forty messages from Europe and the US from individuals who also had laryngectomy and neck radiation and experienced similar symptoms. Most of them received no help from their doctors, who just advised them to get used to living with this condition – much as my doctors had advised me.

I sent a summary of these messages to my physicians, hoping they would start to pay attention to this problem. Some were grateful, and others did not even respond. This was one of many examples I encountered where general practitioners, as well as specialists who care for patients with head and neck cancer, were unaware of serious consequences of radiation of the neck. Fortunately for me, my otolaryngologist sent me to a physical therapist who specializes in rehabilitation of imbalance problems, and she was able to help me to adjust to my symptoms.

Indirect evidence that supports a connection between high blood pressure development and neck radiation – at least in my case – happened three years later. My physical therapist started a series of treatments with a laser beam that was aimed at my stiff and rigid neck muscles. They had become very hard and fibrotic after the radiation and subsequent surgeries I had, and because of this, I had a very limited range of neck motion. The treatment was very successful and reduced the muscle rigidity, and soon I was finally able to move my head from side to side almost to the degree that I was able to do before getting the radiation.

The big surprise was that my blood pressure dropped down significantly after this treatment. This was a new and unexpected result for everyone involved. As a result of this treatment, I was able to gradually discontinue most of the blood pressure medications. I no longer felt light headed or a tendency to faint. Apparently these were a side effect of these medications. The only explanation for the reversal of the high blood pressure was that the reduction in the muscle stiffness decreased the constant pressure these muscles produced on the carotid artery, which contains the delicate blood pressure sensors and regulators. The specialists I told started to believe for the first time that there may be a connection between exposure to radiation and the development of high blood pressure. My radiation oncologist and physical therapist who delivered the treatment were so enthusiastic about the ability of laser therapy to reduce blood pressure that they published a report of my case in a medical journal so that others may also benefit. It was a long struggle, but I was glad my experiences may have opened some eyes and a few new doors to understanding the link between radiation of the neck and high blood pressure side effects.

Even though my sense of taste never returned to its previous capacity, the improvement allowed me to again consume solid and regular food, and I slowly regained the seven pounds that I lost during the course of radiation. I was told by my physicians that my weight loss was minimal, and most patients lose much more weight.

As I was recovering from the radiation, I attempted to drive again. I did not have any objective impairment, but I felt very strange when driving – as if I were a new, inexperienced driver. Oncoming traffic (especially at night) made me very uncomfortable, and I felt as if my sense of orientation was off balance. I avoided driving whenever possible until the feelings of uneasiness disappeared months later.

I was scheduled to have rigorous monthly examination by the Tumor Board, which held a session once a month in the Otolaryngology Clinic in the hospital. This Board was to monitor my recovery from treatment and examine me for any signs of cancer recurrence. Even though the Board consisted of all the specialists needed for follow-up, I soon realized that on each visit, I was only examined by a different junior otolaryngology resident who almost always saw me for the first time and did not know my medical history. Nevertheless, these residents were well meaning and diligent and performed a very thorough otolaryngological examination. After he or she would examine me, an attending staff member examine me as well, often a different attending staff member each time. I never saw any other specialist and realized soon that the fancy title of Tumor Board really stood only for an Otolaryngology Clinic.

I never missed the monthly examination by the Tumor Board. I was told by the otolaryngologists that very close follow-up is crucial to detect cancer recurrence. They warned me that most failures and recurrences are detected within the first two years, and my best chance of surviving was to be vigilant in being reexamined every month during the first year, every two months in the second, and less frequently later – a follow-up schedule I would have to keep for the rest of my life, as my type of cancer can return. These warnings proved very true in my case, and I was fortunate to have complied with these recommendations. I even continued to come for monthly examinations in the second year.

One of the methods used for follow-up were PET and CT scans, which were first performed a few weeks after the end of radiation and then repeated at longer intervals thereafter. These tests take scheduling ahead and expert interpretation. CT scans exposed me to relatively large amounts of X–rays, and PET scans to nuclear radiation, both potentially deleterious. These tests are also difficult to tolerate. The CT required receiving infusion with contrast material, and the PET infusion of radioactively-labeled sugar. The PET required lying still for about an hour, bound to a gurney. However, I was so eager to have these tests done periodically that these issues seemed insignificant to me. When I first had these scans, I was very apprehensive and nervous, because it would be the first time for me to discover if the radiation treatments had been effective and whether or not the whole tumor had been eradicated or spread elsewhere in my body. Unfortunately, this apprehension and worry always preceded future scans, although with time, I began to feel more relaxed and somehow began to believe (falsely, unfortunately) that I may have been cured for good.

I anxiously requested the radiologists to interpret the results as soon as the studies were completed and was disappointed to learn that I had to wait several hours, because the PET scan had to be thoroughly analyzed. I quickly learned about the limitations and pitfalls of these tests because they were unable to detect tumors that were smaller than one to two centimeters. Furthermore, the PET scan, which can only sense high metabolic activity, can raise untoward suspicions in areas of the body that happen to have high metabolic activity for any other reason (such as infection, muscular activity, etc.). Indeed, the second PET scan detected suspicious findings over my right abdominal area, which raised concerns and generated additional studies (gastrointestinal endoscopies and radiological contrast studies). Happily, these all proved negative for cancer. To my great relief, these suspicious findings were never seen again in future PET scans and must have been nonspecific and transitory.

It was a great relief for me to learn that these tests showed no suspicion of recurrence or persistence of the cancer. However, there was still the possibility that the cancer was too small to be detected at this stage. I experienced the cruel reality and limitations of these tests later.

The summer that followed the end of radiation was a long and tedious one of slow recovery and attempts to get back to my feet. My wife and I tried to gain some sense of normality to our lives and celebrated our twenty-fifth wedding anniversary by spending a few days in the beautiful Finger Lakes District in New York State. In spite of the beauty of the area, I found myself spending much time in the hotel room, as the sunlight was irritating to my skin. I felt very tired and unmotivated as my hypothyroidism has not yet been corrected.

In addition to all these medical issues, I had to deal with an unexpected set of events that related to my pending discharge from the US Navy. I was initially very relieved that my discharge and retirement from the Navy were postponed by the Navy's Medical Board, who recommended keeping me on active duty and gave me temporary disability for a year. I was very grateful for the reprieve I got, as it allowed me to concentrate on my treatment and recovery and granted me most needed time for recuperation without having to deal with the difficult transition to regular civilian life. I felt that the system, in its wisdom, worked this time by not abandoning me at a time of extreme need. Unfortunately, I was soon to learn that this assumption was very faulty. The reality was harsher.

The shock came about six weeks after the end of my radiation treatments in the form of a phone message from the Personnel Center of the US Navy, informing me that I needed to attend to my discharge papers. This was a complete surprise to me, as I had received official orders that documented that my discharge was postponed and was not to occur for another ten months. It took several frantic phone calls for me to realize that these orders were mistakenly written and that even though I had been given 100 percent disability, because I was over sixty-five years old, there was no way I could be kept in active duty. My explanation that I was in the middle of a difficult recovery period and that this sudden change in plans would be hard for me fell on deafened or numbed ears. "We are sorry to have made a mistake but, the rules are the rules." I was told. Raising the issues of unfairness and bearing responsibility for an error they made had no impact.

It did not help that I explained that once I learned about the one-year postponement of my discharge from the service, I abandoned looking for work at other places. I explained that I was in the middle of seeking new employment and how I had turned down a lucrative work offer. I went from feeling great gratitude to the Navy to a sense of deep disappointment and disbelief that after over twenty-six years of service, I was cast away at my most desperate time of need and vulnerability. To the difficult process of recovery and recuperation was added the task of fighting the US Navy bureaucracy that eventually forced me to deal with a precipitous discharge.

In my desperation, I consulted Navy Legal Services and even called and wrote to my Congresswoman, to no avail. The Navy lawyers gave me the official party line and just explained the rules, stating that "Even though an initial error was made, it does not obligate the US Navy to follow suit." They advised me, however, that I could delay the process a little by requesting reconsideration of my disability. My Congresswoman's aide wrote a letter of appeal to the Navy on my behalf and demanded an explanation but never even received a response.

I finally became resigned to the inevitable discharge but followed the advice of the Navy lawyers and tried to delay it so that I would feel better and regain some of my energy and stamina. I was fortunate during the period of radiation and the first weeks following it to have had a very understanding Commanding Officer who approved my sick leave and recuperation period. The Commanding Officer plays an important role in the serviceperson's career and must approve any official request.

Unfortunately, things changed a few weeks after the end of my radiation treatment when a new Commanding Officer took over our institute. She was a US Army colonel – a person known for "going by the book" – and did not know me or my work ethic. Even though she was a radiation oncologist by training and should have known what I was going through more than anyone, she was very tough and blatantly refused to understand or consider my difficulties. She was determined to force me to come back to work every day, even though I was physically unable to do so. She repeatedly disregarded sick leave documents written by my doctors that explicitly explained my condition and forced me to call in sick every day that I could not come. This kind of treatment was cruel, humiliating, inhumane, and most demeaning – especially to a person who in all the twenty-six years of service rarely used any sick leave and showed up for work at least ten hours a day, including many weekends and holidays.

She was determined to prevent me from going through the appeal process and disapproved my legal requests for due process whenever she could. Due to her active efforts, I was unable to exhaust the appeal process or even get a terminal discharge leave and was forced to retire five months earlier. She asked me to vacate my office in advance of my discharge, even though I was at the peak of my hypothyroidism and was very exhausted and breathless. I vacated my office despite my difficult physical condition. I got some help from fellow workers in carrying the heavy boxes to my car, but I had to perform the difficult task of dismantling and reviewing all my files and records that I accumulated over a twenty-six year period. I had to bring all these files home, where I unpacked them myself because the colonel disapproved any assistance or the use of a government car.

There are no words that can describe the difficulties, aggravation, humiliation, and disrespect I endured during this period because of the misdeeds and pure inhumanity of a single person that just happened to be my Commanding Officer. She seemed to be most resourceful in making the process more difficult and demeaning than it already was. It was not enough that I had to struggle with cancer and its sequella, but I also had to bear inhuman hardships inflicted on me by a person who was supposed to help me.

It was a most disappointing and disheartening way to end more than twenty-six years of military service after receiving several Defense Meritorious Service Medals for exceptional meritorious service from the Armed Forces of the United States. I devoted those years to contribute milestone achievements for the treatment and prevention of serious infections in military personnel, yet the same courtesy was not imparted to me upon my exit from the service.

Prior to my retirement, I needed to be thoroughly examined by professionals at the Veterans Affairs (VA) system to determine any disability I might have. Even though I had completed two years of fellowship in that system thirty years earlier before I joined the US Navy, I had become skeptical about its efficacy. It was a refreshing experience to deal with the system at the local VA hospital. I was touched by the care, compassion, and gratitude for my military service that I felt at each level. I felt comradeship with the patients there which I had not previously experienced as a physician in that facility. This was because I had experienced the military service just as they did, and was humbled by the serious illness I had to live through. I was also very impressed by the excellence, knowledge, and professionalism I encountered among the medical personnel in the VA Hospital. It made me feel better about my future medical options, and I felt I could rely on the VA system should I ever need to.

I retired from the US Navy about six month after the end of the radiation course and had an official retirement ceremony a month later. It was a very moving ceremony attended by my close family, friends, and the entire institute. I received my third Defense Meritorious Service Medal and many letters of appreciation, including one from the Unites States president (who is the Commander in Chief), and a USA flag that had been flown over the US Capitol in Washington DC, boxed up beautifully with my awards and medals. My colleagues placed in the box my picture in front of a camouflaged ambulance marked with the Star of David, wearing the Israeli Defense Forces Uniform – a picture taken a short time before the Yom Kippur War in 1973. This farewell box symbolized my lifelong service to both countries, which I always felt was a continuous effort to contribute to the security of each. I had the opportunity to graciously summarize my entire Navy career and listen to very personal presentations made by my colleagues and friends. It was definitely a gracious ending to my long service.

Even so, my retirement day was bittersweet. During my long naval service, I always felt that I was part of an extended family. I felt cared for by other Navy personal at all levels. This feeling of belonging was very real for me, especially when I needed medical care, and mostly when I was admitted to the Naval Hospital. I felt more vulnerable at this time knowing that I had cancer and was unsure whether I was cured. I was now in uncharted waters on my own and had no idea how the future would play out. I had many questions in my mind, constantly unsure about the quality of care I would receive as a retiree. I was comforted by assurances that my medical care would stay the same.

The future would show me that, overall, the quality of service by military hospitals remained almost the same. However, I lost the priority enlisted personal have in pharmacy and laboratory services, and many clinics closed their doors to me as a retiree. On the other hand, I gained the freedom for the first time to seek medical care elsewhere because I was entitled to Medicare and VA services, and my government health coverage permitted me to get medical care in the private sector. In reality, I chose to stick with the military system whenever I could, mostly because of its excellence, and also because I was used to it and knew and trusted many of the providers there. However, the freedom to venture outside government hospitals was a right I also learned to appreciate in the future.

Chapter 6. Am I cured?

Once I was officially discharged from the Navy, I had mixed feelings of relief and emptiness. On the one hand, I had the freedom of planning my own days and traveled freely without the need to report my whereabouts, request permission to travel, or miss work. On the other hand, I had become so used to these restrictions that they became second nature for me. For so many years, every time I was about to take or return from leave or official travel, I had to call the front desk of my command and register my departure or return with the on-duty officer. It was a difficult routine to break.

What I realized was that over the years I had actually even learned to like the obligation to report my whereabouts; it gave me a feeling that I belonged to a big family and that I was an important part of that organization, essential enough that I may be needed at any time. Indeed, there had been occasions where I was contacted while I was away to provide essential assistance that only I could deliver. The reality, of course, is that accountability is a mandatory requirement for all members of the military, whatever their position or responsibility. Also, as a physician in charge of patients or on call, I had to always carry a beeper or a cell phone so I could be contacted should I be needed. Suddenly, all of these obligations – these important duties – were just gone. I was not essential for anyone except my family.

I also missed the many opportunities my employment allowed me. It enabled me to conduct clinical and laboratory research, be on national committees, control a research budget, and take care of patients. *Whatever I do now will be only as a volunteer*, I thought, *and that depends on the willingness of others to accept me as such.* I also lost access to all that I had built for so many years: the research laboratory with all its sophisticated instruments, the office equipment, and the support system that made my professional life possible. These included the computer, all the graphic, editorial, and administrative support, the office space that contained all my files and records, and the financial support I received to travel and participate in professional meetings.

Suddenly, I had the freedom to dress any way I wanted and no longer had to put on my military uniform. For the first time in almost three decades, I had to make a daily decision how to dress. I no longer had to salute or do thing "by the book" as I had previously done.

The military uniform I had been forced to wear had been a relief because I did not have to worry about what to wear. I grew up in Israel in a period of austerity, and the cultural emphasis was on what you did and who you were – not how you dressed. I had gone to a high school that required a uniform dress code, one of the few in the country at that time, emphasizing the school's motto of simplicity and modesty and serving as a great equalizer that erased class and family earning differences. Even though I came from a working-class family where my father was a welder and my mother a seamstress, I felt equal to my classmates who came from wealthier families with parents who were in business or working as lawyers or physicians. At my high school, the uniforms helped students concentrate on their studies rather than on how they dress. Wearing a uniform had long been a custom for me, even before I entered the military, and now, at my retirement, even this changed.

In addition to the security and comfortable familiarity with it, I missed wearing the uniform because it represented my status as an officer, and as a person who serves his country. On the other hand, not needing to wear the Navy uniform any longer was somewhat of a relief, for when you are donning the uniform, you tend to stand out in the crowd, and your conduct and demeanor are always being watched to be sure you are representing the US Navy well. It is difficult to relax under such scrutiny.

Wearing a uniform had also been somewhat difficult for me because I had never been able to dress quite right. I never paid too much attention to the fine details of the uniform, in contrast to other military personal. It got me into trouble on several occasions, earning me several remarks from military commanders. Part of my difficulties came from my previous experience while serving in the Israeli military during a period when the dress code was more relaxed. My recent years of service there were in the military reserves where the dress code was even looser than in the regular army. Emphasis there was on performance rather than on uniform and appearance, so I had become a bit lax in that department.

Even though I did not like saluting when I was in service, I get satisfaction and feel gratitude for being recognized as an officer when military personal salute me whenever I show my military retiree identification card at the gates of military installation. Similarly I feel grateful when I am thanked for my service to the country when I visit the Veteran Administration clinics.

Prior to being diagnosed with cancer, I considered working as a civilian in the research institute where I spent the past two and a half decades or seeking meaningful employment at another location such as the NIH or Food and Drug Administration. However, my perspective changed. My time was filled more and more by medical problems that continuously emerged and the follow-up appointments needed to correct them. I even considered spending a few months in Israel, where I could volunteer to teach and work in a university hospital or a community clinic where there is shortage of physicians. However, I felt reluctant to leave my "safe" environment where I had easy access to medical care, including the physicians who knew me and other support systems. I also felt physically weak, had less energy, and required more resting time than before. Not having any work obligations made it easier for me to accommodate my activities according to my current abilities.

Staying home alone all day was difficult after a while. I was warned that for most people, retirement and inactivity are detrimental to one's health and psychological well-being. I found this even more difficult after being diagnosed with cancer. I realized that I could quickly slide into depression and despair and that I needed to actively prevent this. I realized that in order to avoid confinement in my home, I needed to seek out contacts and activities that suited me best, and no one else was going to do it for me. It was up to me to change the situation, and I needed to be proactive.

Even though I accepted the offer to continue to work at the research institution as a volunteer in the capacity of a visiting scientist, I was reluctant to spend much time there, mostly because of the difficult time I had with the commanding officer. However, I did not want to abandon that opportunity completely. I had worked more than twenty five years at that institute and felt that the work done there was very important and essential for patients' well-being and national and international security. I knew that my input was essential for research progress and very much wanted to continue to contribute to its success. Knowing that there was no one else that could fill the gap created when I retired, I tried to overcome the personal insult I felt and continued to visit and consult. However, I kept my visits short and limited them to contact with my previous colleagues, with whom I discussed ongoing experiments and plans for future research. It was very gratifying to see that I could still contribute to the work and that the projects I had to abandon when I retired were efficiently carried on by others.

I continued to participate in medical rounds at the two local military hospitals and provide advice as I had previously done. I also spent more time as a teaching faculty member at a university hospital in town. These activities kept me connected to my professional life and allowed me to continue to contribute to patient care and education of the residents and students. The only difference was that I no longer had direct responsibility for patient care or research activities, and my advice could be accepted or rejected according to its value and merits. However, I felt appreciation from those involved, which gave me great satisfaction because I realized that my direct involvement made a difference. It was gratifying to realize that should I have not come to medical rounds that day, patient care would have missed an important element that I was able to deliver – or that the residents and medical students would not have gained knowledge that I provided. It was also rewarding to be able to continue to draw on the wealth of information and experience I had in research and patient care in order to assist my colleagues. Because of these activities, I needed to stay current in medicine by reading medical and scientific literature and attending educational lectures.

I also continued to be invited to give lectures locally as well as nationally, served as a reviewer for professional journals, edited two medical journals, and worked on the fourth edition of a textbook I wrote. All of these activities kept me busy and involved to the extent that I did not even feel that I had truly retired. This was a positive way of adapting to my new situation. At times, I almost forgot that I had been diagnosed with cancer, even though I was very much aware that it could come back at any time. As time progressed and months passed without any sign of cancer recurrence or spreading, I started to feel more and more confident that I had been cured.

I was willing (for the first time in months) to consider planning for the future rather than expecting an impending end. When my wife first discussed the need to renovate our old house, I was unwilling to even consider it – mainly because I was not sure how long I had left to live. I asked myself *Why spend the little time I have to live in construction and dust?* and *Why does my wife need more space after I die? She will probably sell the house and move to a smaller place afterwards anyway,* I thought. I initially did not share these fears and true reasons for my reluctance to do the renovations with her, opting to keep the morbid, pessimistic thoughts and fears to myself. Eventually, as she kept bringing up the subject, I shared my true reasons with her. I told her that I preferred to wait some more time, perhaps until the two years were up when the probability of cancer recurrence dropped significantly. I tried to drag my feet any time she brought the topic up, so as to delay the actual decision until the magic date. I also felt too tired to add the additional burden of living in a house during renovation.

In addition to the real need that existed to renovate our house, what also motivated my wife was her wish to go on with life and move away from the painful memories of the cancer and its aftermath. I believe that, at that time, she may have felt that by fixing what was broken in the house, she was able to correct something belonging to us that needed mending. Cancer cannot always be completely controlled, and chronic illnesses do not go away, but old houses can be repaired. She needed something she could control and fix because my cancer had made her feel helpless and powerless.

In her mind, something new and positive would emerge after we concluded the renovation. She also wished that by improving our living conditions, our lives would become better and more enjoyable in the future. In some symbolic way, fixing the house was like fixing my future ... my wife's "If you build it, they will come" wish. I was more skeptical than she and had an underlying fear that my saga was not yet over. I was afraid that the cancer would return and wanted to wait and see if it did. Unfortunately, I was right in my premonitions. However, as I was approaching the two-year mark, I was willing to consider the renovation because I felt more and more confident about my health. We started actively planning for the renovation and began interviewing architects and visited several recently renovated homes in our neighborhood.

That summer, we took a very enjoyable two-week trip to Croatia and had a great experience traveling throughout the country. We relished the beautiful coastline, picturesque islands, nature reserves, antique cities, and local dishes. The only limitations I had were the results of the long-term effects of the radiation. I had to avoid eating spicy food because my sensitivity to taste had intensified. I had to consume only moist food because I had reduced production of saliva. The recently discovered hypertension also made me avoid salty food as much as possible. I purposefully postponed the PET and CT scans I was to have before the trip until after our return from our vacation. I thought to myself, *If there are going to be any suspicious findings or other "bad news" discovered by these scans, I will at least have a nice trip to remember.* I simply did not want to cancel the trip in case there were any ominous results.

I was bothered in the summer months (about a year after my radiation treatment) by a nagging pain in the right side of my throat, similar to the kind of pain I had before my initial tumor was diagnosed. I repeatedly informed the otolaryngologists about the pain on each of my monthly follow-up examinations. Even though they examined me thoroughly and routinely performed endoscopy of my upper airways, they did not see any lesion that suggested a return of the cancer. They kept reassuring me that since there were no cancer-like findings, the pain was most likely due to irritation of the irradiated airway mucosa by reflux of stomach acid. Even after they increased the acid reducing medication I was taking, the pain did not subside. I was relieved when the CT and PET scans of the painful area came back negative. Unfortunately, I was reminded a few days later that these scans are imperfect.

Chapter 7. Cancer Returns

I was sitting in the Otolaryngology Clinic with an endoscopic tube sliding down my throat when everything changed. It was on a routine monthly examination twenty months after the initial cancer was detected. As I had been doing in all recent routine monthly visits, I told the otolaryngology resident about the persistent pain in my right throat. The resident who had never seen me before performed a thorough examination that included endoscopy of the upper airways. What he did differently that time during the endoscopy, which I later learned, helped him look much deeper in my throat. He asked me to blow air into my closed mouth during the procedure. The resident told me some time later that he routinely performed this maneuver, because this is how he was taught. Halfway through the process, he stopped to share his findings with a medical student that accompanied him. When he finished, he looked at me with concerned eyes and told me, "I have seen something suspicious and need to have the senior attending physician look at it as well." Within a few minutes, he was joined by the attending that also looked down my throat and nodded his head in agreement. I sensed something had happened. *Things are not right anymore. Has the cancer come back?*

The resident and attending told me that they observed a suspicious looking 2 x 1.2 centimeter ulcer unlike the lesion seen before, which was a polyp. The observation was also confirmed by another staff member, Dr. Strom, who had just completed a fellowship in head and neck cancer. They all explained to me that this structure was suspicious looking and needed to be biopsied and examined by a pathologist to find out if it was cancerous.

I tried to argue and ameliorate the bad news by asking them if this ulcer could have been caused by stomach acid irritation or was the result of the radiation I had received. I was wishing they would give me a good differential diagnosis rather than the grim possibility of cancer.

"How could this be cancer? Cancer usually does not cause pain," I insisted. "I just had a negative PET and CT scans." The look in the doctors' eyes did not give me any reassurance. I sensed that they could not give me any comforting options and only suspected the worse. There was nothing positive they could tell me until the biopsy results were examined. I could not argue my way out of this and had to wait.

The waiting for the biopsy, which was scheduled a few days later, seemed very long and hard. I shared the news with my wife but tried to present it in the least ominous fashion and underplayed the potential for cancer recurrence by describing the suspicious finding as an ulcer which needed to be examined only as a precaution.

As I had previously done, on the day of the scheduled biopsy I arrived at the hospital alone. Prior to being wheeled to the operating room, I again met Dr. Strom, the staff cancer specialist who promised to take good care of me and let me know the results as soon as possible. I tried to remain optimistic and hoped to hear good news when I woke up. I repeatedly told myself, *It is really unlikely that I have cancer again because the original one was detected at a very early stage, and I received large doses of radiation that should have eliminated all remaining tumor.*

All seemed like a repeat of what had happened to me before. I was brought down to the chilly operating room where I started to shiver a little, again due to the cool temperature and my anxiety. I asked for a blanket, which made me feel a little warmer. The waiting was short, and I was put to sleep within a few minutes.

I woke up some time later in the recovery room feeling intense pain in my throat, which was to be expected after the diagnostic procedure. A short time later, Dr. Strom walked in and delivered the bad news: the initial assessment of the biopsy showed the same kind of cancer I had before. Since I was still partially under the influence of the anesthetics, I could not fully digest and experience the entire impact of what he had just told me. The effects of medication made the news less scary and easier to hear. He also briefly discussed what the next steps would be, which included the surgical options he was planning. However, I could not recall the exact details of his plan, which he repeated again in the coming days. Realizing that I was still sedated, he told me he would return later and asked me to come to his clinic the next morning, where he would outline the surgical and therapeutic strategy.

The knowledge that there was a planned course of action made me feel that I was in good and caring hands. When I finally came back to myself and faced my wife, who came later to take me home, I slowly began to fully digest the ominous news and all its dire implications.

Many questions ran through my mind. *How is it possible that cancer returned?* My original cancer was caught very early and was very small. Furthermore, it was supposed to have been completely eliminated by the intense radiation I had received. *How come it was not seen at an earlier date by my doctors?* I saw them every month and repeatedly complained about the pain for the past five months. This tumor could not have grown to its present size overnight. *Why did they miss it before?* I was examined by a radiation oncologist just three weeks earlier who had seen no abnormality when he performed an endoscopic examination of my upper airway. This specialist confessed to me later that he actually did not look down into the area where the new cancer was found because his instrument broke down during his examination. Although I was angry at his failure to do the test appropriately, which delayed the diagnosis of the malignancy, I had deep appreciation for his kindness, care, and compassion and kept returning to him for my care. I also did not appreciate that radiation oncologists are less experienced in performing endoscopic examination than otolaryngologists. As it became clear to me later, no one had used the air puffing maneuver that the resident who discovered the recurrence performed. I couldn't help but wonder, *Are the doctors to blame for the delay in diagnosis? Will this delay lead to failure of therapy because the cancer has already spread?*

My belief that I was finally cured was suddenly shattered. I was facing an uncertain future, impending surgeries, and had to deal again with the possibility of an approaching death.

Why is this happening to me? Why am I the unfortunate one who fails treatment? What kind of deficient immune system do I have that allows such a failure? Did I not do everything right? I came to all the follow-up monthly visits and did all the follow-up scans.

These are not fears I shared with my spouse. I told my wife about the bad news using a matter-of-fact tone without panicking or showing signs of desperation in spite of my own questioning mind. I briefly shared with her the outline of the surgical plan that I heard about earlier. I attempted to convey to her a sense that I was in good hands and that the physicians taking care of me knew what they were doing, cared about me, and were going to do whatever was necessary to get rid of my cancer. We waited for Dr. Strom to return as he had promised, and when he did, he explained the general plan also to my wife. He reminded us to come to his office the next morning so that we could discuss the situation further when I was more awake and had more time to absorb the news.

I returned back home and into a new reality and sense of hope. It was good and reassuring to know that we were going to the doctor again to learn more about the treatment plan.

We were in the doctor's office early the next morning. Dr. Strom spent more than an hour outlining his surgical plans and explained all the procedures he would employ using an anatomical model of the neck. He was a very kind, warm, caring person and conveyed a sense of security and reassurance that we both badly needed. "What is necessary," he explained," is to entirely remove the cancerous lesion as well as the cervical lymph nodes at the right side and replace the surgically resectioned area with a flap of tissue that will be obtained from your thigh or shoulder region." He was planning to save my larynx and vocal cords if at all possible. "However," he forewarned, "the extent of how much tissue is going to be removed is impossible to predict until the actual surgery, when biopsies of the surrounding tissues will be performed." These biopsies would allow him to know when the entire cancer had been removed.

He assured us that both he and the rest of the surgical team were very experienced in this type of surgery and had all the equipment needed to perform it. He told us that he had recently completed a fellowship in this area at one of the most prestigious cancer centers in the country, where he had done or assisted in numerous such operations. I would undergo a two-stage procedure. The first surgery would be to prepare a piece of tissue from my shoulder that would form the flap that would be transplanted a week later into my neck during the second surgery to replace the tissue he was going to remove. The resection of the tumor and removal of the cervical lymph glands were also to be done on the second surgery.

"It is quite possible," Dr. Strom explained, "although unlikely in my opinion, that a much greater area including the vocal cords will have to be removed." I had to be ready to face the possibility that I might not be able to speak again afterwards. It all depended how extensive the cancer was and, consequently, how much tissue had to be removed. He estimated the length of the surgery to be nine to thirteen hours, after which I would be sent to an intensive care unit (ICU) for a day; and the total length of my hospitalization he predicted would be about ten days. Following surgery, I was to receive intravenous fluids and be fed with liquid food by a tube through my nose until the post-surgical swelling subsided and the transplanted flap was fully integrated and healed. That was estimated to range between fourteen to twenty-one days.

We talked about the date of the surgery and set a tentative date for fourteen days later. I was very eager to have the surgery as early as possible. I wanted the cancer out of my body as soon as possible because I believed that my chances for survival were better if the tumor was removed before it had a chance to spread to other parts of my body. However, an earlier date was not possible; it was the holiday season, and many staff members were away on vacation. The hospital was not fully staffed, and elective surgeries were postponed. Furthermore, some essential members of the surgical team, including Dr. Cooper, the Head of the Department of Otolaryngology at the Army hospital in town who was to assist Dr. Strom, were on vacation and did not even know about my case. To my request to expedite the process, he responded by explaining "I understand your concerns, but generally, this cancer does not spread rapidly. It tends first to seed the local cervical lymph nodes, which may halt its general dissemination to the liver and lungs for a while." He assured me that a two week delay was safe and that my outcome would not be compromised by this delay. I still wanted the tumor out of my body as soon as possible.

Hearing about these options in detail was overwhelming and hard for me to completely appreciate and integrate. We had numerous questions but could not think about everything. At this time, I wanted to be cured and rid myself of the cancer so much that I was ready to pay any price in discomfort, pain, or loss of functions such as eating or speaking. All these consequences paled in comparison with the option of dying from cancer. Even though many of these side effects were described to me on several occasions and by numerous individuals, nothing could prepare me to how they actually felt once I experienced and endured them.

Some of my questions were "Is this cancer a recurrence of the old one, or is it a new tumor? Did the radiation treatment I received fail since the area where the new lesion was found was also irradiated? This area received less amount of radiation than the site of the cancer, but was it enough to destroy any budding tumor?"

"These questions can not be answered at present," the specialist explained, "but maybe they can be answered during the upcoming surgery. However," he proceeded, "in my opinion, since the new finding was about two inches away from the original one, it may represent a new cancer rather than a recurrence of the old one." It felt better hearing this response because it meant that my chances of recovery were going to be as good as before. He stressed that my cancer was still small and most likely could be successfully removed in its entirety.

He also explained that head and neck cancer recur in about thirty percent of patients in the first five years after the tumor is diagnosed, and most recurrences are in the first two years. *I guess I am one of the unfortunate ones that fall into this group,* I said to myself. *Why can I not be an average patient?*

I was uncertain how competent and experienced the members of my surgical team were, wondering if I should seek treatment elsewhere, perhaps in a more prestigious institution or find more experienced surgeons. However, at that stage, I was so overwhelmed by the news and seemingly had a caring, competent physician taking care of me that I did not dwell on this issue for long. Since the operations I was having were not unusual and had been done numerous times at that hospital, I felt that there were sufficient experience and skills there to provide me with the optimal care.

I also felt more secure having the surgery at the hospital where I had worked for the past twenty-seven years because I knew so many doctors and staff. This was the place where I had all my medical and surgical care done before, and I was generally very pleased with it. Also, the sense of camaraderie and care I felt at all levels made me feel that I was not just a patient, but a member of a large family where everyone would do their best for me. This was indeed a unique sensation that I could not feel anywhere else.

I did check around a little and consulted several members of the hospital staff about my surgeons, and they all gave me rave reviews about them. It reassured me that I was doing the right thing by not looking elsewhere. Furthermore, I did not have the strength to start looking around the country for alternatives. It was also appealing for me to have a date set for surgery. Looking for another location would cause further delay, with all its potential devastating consequences.

Once we left the doctor's office I decided to see for myself the pathological specimens. As when I first learned about the diagnosis of cancer about twenty months earlier, I needed to see it to believe it. I bid my wife goodbye and walked over to the pathological laboratories and asked to speak with the pathologist. I wanted again to "look the evil directly in the eyes." I needed visual confirmation to truly believe the news.

And there was no doubt – it was the same cancer. The pathologist compared the new specimen with the older one, and the two looked almost identical. I was wondering if my type of malignancy could be induced by papilloma virus, because I had recently read about such an association. However, this was not determined at that stage. I asked the pathologist if such a test could be made, because the prognosis of patients with virus-induced cancer is slightly better; she promised to do that when the new cancer was surgically removed. The pathologist I spoke with was frank and honest. I met her in the hospital corridors a few months later, and after inquiring about my health, she had tears in her eyes. I had no idea why, but I felt that she really cared and sensed my pain and struggle.

I walked over to the radiological diagnostic office to rereview my recent CT scan with the expert who had interpreted it before. I thought, *How could such an expert who is a known expert in the field have missed the cancer?* I showed him the site of the tumor in the scans, and only after that was he able to notice minimal ulcer-like indentation. "Even this," he told me "is within normal variability seen in healthy individuals." This was a shocking realization to me, that even such a sophisticated diagnostic tool has its limitations and that there is no substitute to visual examination if it is possible. It was a vivid illustration that there is no test available today that can detect early developing cancer.

When I returned home, we had to face the task of conveying the news to our children, who did not yet know about the recent development or biopsy results, and if and how to tell other individuals about it. This time, my reaction to the situation was different, and I had no objection to sharing the news and my medical condition with others. This was not something I could hide or deny anymore, especially since I was going to be hospitalized for a long time and might not speak the same again thereafter. This illness and its consequences were going to affect our lives in such a major way that this could no longer be kept private. This must have been a relief for my wife and children, who could now share their feelings and difficulties with others and get support and assistance.

Breaking the news to the children was not easy, but it was less difficult than it was the first time. My wife and I did it together and in person to all of them except to my oldest daughter, who resides in California, whom we had to inform by phone. Since the rest of my children lived in New York City, we traveled there over the weekend and shared the news with each of them separately. We asked those we told first to wait until we shared the news with their siblings. Each of them had to be told in a way that we felt was suitable for them. We did our best to deliver the news in a fashion that was optimistic and stressed the potential for recovery. It was, however, a very difficult and emotionally challenging task.

The weekend we spent in New York was a very cold and windy one. The atmosphere was gloomy and sad, similar to the weather around us. The only one who was cheerful and happy was my four-year-old granddaughter, who was oblivious to the situation and did not fully appreciate what was going on. We tried to enjoy ourselves the best we could by going to the park, a children's science museum, and to restaurants. However, the freezing air and the impending difficulties and uncertainty made enjoying these activities very difficult. I felt this was going to be the last weekend our family was going to have together before embarking on the long and difficult road that was waiting for all of us, and this fear robbed me of some of the joy of being together.

A few days later, I spoke with my surgeon again, and he informed me that the hospital Tumor Board approved his treatment plan, with a slight change. After discussing the plans with Dr. Cooper, they decided that they would perform the reconstruction of the larynx with a graft obtained from the skin and subcutaneous tissues of my thigh instead of my shoulder, and all of this would be done in one operation. I was pleased with the news, as it meant having to endure only one surgery.

The whole holiday season passed without any feeling of celebration or relaxation. There was a feeling of uncertainty and fear of the unknown in the upcoming year looming in the air at all times. I was robotic, doing my daily chores, and did my best to conclude all unfinished work and tasks, including manuscripts I had to write or edit, fixing the house, and paying bills. I did not know if or when I would be back from the hospital and how I would feel. This was indeed going to be one of the most difficult years of my life.

Chapter 8. What is the Best Surgery?

A week before the scheduled surgery, I was informed by my surgeon, Dr. Strom, that there was again a change in the surgical plan. He had further discussions with Dr. Cooper, the Head of the Otolaryngology Department at the Army Hospital, who, after learning more about the details of my condition, changed his opinion about what would be the best surgical approach. He now believed that a less extensive and invasive treatment was possible. This would achieve the same goal of removing the tumor, but would also preserve my larynx and other neck structures so I would not need any reconstruction of my neck. This would be possible if the cancer was cut out by a laser instrument introduced from my mouth into my upper airways. The procedure would be guided by an endoscope and would allow removal of the cancer without cutting through my neck. My right neck lymph glands would, however, be removed by open dissection. There would still be an option to revert to the previous surgical plan if the surgeons would not be able to remove the entire tumor by laser. There was also a possibility that an even more extensive surgery would be required involving complete excision of the larynx and the vocal cords, which would involve more reconstruction of the upper airways. However, these options would be decided upon only during the planned operation or later, depending on the pathological evaluation that would determine the extent of the cancer spread.

When I asked for more details, Dr. Strom explained that he would have preferred to perform the more extensive surgery, but deferred his opinion to his more senior partner. He also informed me that it was up to me to consent to the new approach, and if I did not feel confident about using the laser to remove the cancer, they would revert to the original plan.

"The advantage of the laser approach," he explained, "is that it is a less complicated procedure requiring much less surgical, hospitalization, and recovery time. Furthermore, your ability to eat and speak will only be compromised for a few weeks. In contrast, the more extensive surgery may leave you with permanent swallowing difficulties and a tendency to aspirate food into your lungs. The disadvantage of the laser approach is that the ability to visualize the tumor and remove it in its entirety is not as good compared with the conventional one. However," he continued, "the follow-up after laser surgery needs to be more intense and will require inspection of your upper airways for recurrences every few months under general anesthesia."

He set another meeting in two days, and Dr. Cooper, who was still on vacation, would be coming back to join us. During that conference, my wife and I would be able to get more clarification and ask more questions.

The change of plans was surprising to me. I was mentally prepared to undergo the extensive surgery and did not even realize that there was a less invasive option. I was naturally interested and happy to hear about the new plan. However, I was afraid that this less invasive surgery might not lead to complete recovery – a cure. The removal of cancer by laser was a new technology and not yet fully accepted or practiced. I was afraid that there might not be sufficient proof that it was as effective as the conventional approach. As a physician, I had seen new therapeutic fads come and go over time, and the patients who tried them paid the price of getting inappropriate therapy. We anxiously waited for the upcoming meeting and prepared numerous questions. I started to educate myself about the utility of laser surgery for throat cancer but was overwhelmed by the complexity of the topic.

We came back for the meeting where, with the assistance of a neck and mouth anatomical model, the surgeons elaborated on their plans. They assured us that they were going to lead a well-experienced surgical team that could perform the operation. The estimated time required for the laser and lymph gland removal would be about eight to nine hours, whereas the longer procedure would require up to thirteen. "The reason so much time is required," they explained, "is that every stage of the surgery will be guided by a microscopical examination of the specimens obtained during the procedure by a pathologist."

They proceeded to go over the order of events. After putting me to sleep, an endoscope would be inserted down my mouth through which the cancerous lesion could be visualized. That lesion would be cut out in its entirety using a laser beam and sent to the pathological laboratory. To insure that there was no cancer left in me, a series of biopsies would be obtained around the excision site, as well as other sites in the hypopharynx, including the site where I had cancer twenty-one months prior. These tissues would be frozen and immediately inspected in the operating room by a pathologist. If no cancerous cells were observed in the margins around the excised tumor, this would signify that the entire tumor had been successfully removed. However, if cancer cells were seen, more tissue would be removed from that area, and again biopsies beyond that location would be examined under the microscope. This sequence of procedures would be repeated until all the cancer was removed. They cautioned me that, "although the pathological examination of the frozen specimens done at the operating room is a rapid way of establishing a diagnosis, it is an imperfect technique that requires confirmation using a better one which may require up to one week."

If cancer was discovered at other areas, the use of laser would be abandoned, and my neck would be surgically opened to perform an extensive removal of the cancerous area or the entire larynx; and subsequent reconstruction would be required. I would find out what had transpired and if I would be able to speak again only when I woke up from anesthesia. The doctors assured me that "your waiting family will be immediately informed about the pathological findings and the required surgery."

Should partial or complete removal of the larynx be done, I was going to have a tracheotomy, where my trachea would be disconnected from my throat and opened up into my neck. This would allow me to breathe around the operated area, which would be swollen and might bleed. If only partial resection was done, the tracheotomy would be temporary and would stay in place only for a few weeks. However, if my entire larynx was removed, it would be permanent.

After the operation, I would be admitted to the Surgical Intensive Care Unit (SICU) for a period of twenty-four to forty-eight hours and then moved to the surgical ward. I would receive my medication intravenously and be fed by a tube inserted into my stomach through my nose. This mode of feeding would continue until the surgical sites healed and the swelling decreased, which might take from ten to fourteen days. Since I previously had extensive neck radiation, the expected healing time would be longer than usual.

The quality of my life afterwards would depend on the kind of surgery I would have. If only laser was used, I would have minimal long-term effects, but if an extensive resection was needed, I might have swallowing difficulties and be susceptible to food aspiration into my lungs. If my vocal cords were to be removed, I would need to use alternative ways to speak – such as using an artificial larynx (called Electro-Larynx), a tracheo-esophageal voice prosthesis, or laryngeal speech. I would be guided by a Speech and Language Pathologist (SLP) who would work with me and assist me in choosing and using the method of speech I selected. If my vocal cords were to be removed, the surgeons were going to create a tracheo-esophageal puncture (TEP); a connection between my trachea and my esophagus which would house the voice prosthesis.

I was overwhelmed by the substance and amount of information I was getting. There was so much to hear, absorb, understand, and internalize. Most of what I heard was too abstract and difficult to appreciate. Listening to all the information, however, helped me prepare for the unknown future. But as I was to realize later, there was so much more to understand and appreciate. These things were not said or could never be truly explained. I had to learn how it felt by living through these experiences and coping with them. I wish now there had been a way to be better prepared for what was to come.

My surgeons highlighted the positive aspect of achieving cure with a minimalist procedure and stressed, "among the other advantages, the preservation of your vocal cords will allow you to continue to give lectures and communicate with your peers." I was not able to appreciate then the importance of preserving one's natural voice.

"Do whatever is medically needed," I responded, "and should it be required to remove my vocal cords, just go ahead." I signed my surgical consent form on that day to allow them to do whatever they deemed necessary. Although the surgeons offered to wake me up from my anesthesia should a decision be needed to be made, I gave up that option. By signing those documents, I gave up my right to choose what should be done during the surgery, but since I would be anaesthetized, I trusted my surgeons would do what was best for me. The bottom line: I wanted to insure that all the cancerous tissues were removed.

My wife and I tried to ask as many questions as we could think of. There were so many more that we did not think about at that time, so many more issues needed clarification and explanation. It was all quite a lot to grasp at once.

At the end of the hour-long session, we felt that we were in the hands of very dedicated and responsible doctors who would do the best in their abilities to get me cured. I was, however, unsure about the best surgery I should have – the laser or the conventional one.

In the following days, I tried to educate myself about head and neck cancer surgery by reading selected manuscripts and books, information I could glean from the Internet, and by talking with colleagues. However, it was difficult for me to stay calm, impartial, and objective.

I felt that I needed to be vigilant and proactive to find out for myself what the best treatment for me was. This was my life at stake. Since my surgeons admitted that they would leave the final decision to me, I felt that I had to get the best information I could.

Since my surgery was postponed for additional twelve days, I decided to use the time to get the advice of other experts around the world. I started by searching the medical literature to identify individuals who published manuscripts on head and neck cancer in general and those who used laser technology to remove cancer. I learned through reading the literature and contacts with specialists that the laser approach to remove neck cancer (thereby replacing the more extensive procedure) was pioneered in Germany about twenty years prior and that most of the advances in that field were made there. The laser procedure was infrequently used in the USA, where the traditional approach was the standard of care. However, there were several centers in the USA that were performing large numbers of laser surgeries. These were in Phoenix, Arizona; Jacksonville, Florida; and St. Louis, Missouri. I also identified through the Internet the names of personnel in the departments of otolaryngology at the major cancer centers in the USA. I planned to write to otolaryngologists who worked in these centers.

I prepared a general letter introducing myself and my medical background, told them about my medical history and the types of surgeries offered to me, and asked for their advice in choosing the most appropriate one. I emailed this letter to about twenty physicians:

Dear Dr. …:

I am an infectious disease physician (with special interest in head and neck infections) and very much enjoyed reading your recent article on…

Unfortunately, these issues have recently become a major personal problem for me as I developed a recurrence of my hypopharyngeal cancer. I would very much appreciate your advice concerning the surgical options that have been placed before me. As an expert in the field, your opinion would be most helpful to me.

I learned last week that my throat cancer (first diagnosed twenty months ago as moderate to well-differentiated midline hypopharyngeal squamous cell carcinoma, T1. L0, M0) had returned at a different place in the hypopharynx in the right pitiform sinus (now T1-2, L0, M 0). It is 1.8x2.2 cm. PET and CT scans were negative.

I am due now to undergo extensive surgery for removal and grafting in ten days at ... Hospital. Radiation is no longer an option, as I received a full course for the original tumor.

The planned surgery by Dr. [Strom] was to do right partial pharyngectomy and neck dissection, pharyngeal reconstruction (free flap), tracheotomy, and possible partial laryngectomy. He is going to do it with Dr. [Cooper] who is very experienced in flap reconstruction. However, Dr. [Cooper] is now inclined to forego the extensive resection and remove the tumor endoscopically and do also the neck dissection. The benefits will be no need for flaps and quicker recovery. He has the equipment and training to do endoscopic removal of the cancer.

I wonder if, in your opinion, this endoscopic approach is reliable and at least equally effective in removal of the cancer with safe margins.

I would very much appreciate your opinion and advice. Is this approach worthwhile, or would the conventional approach be better?

Thanks so much,

The responses to the letter were quick and universal. They were split between those who preferred the traditional surgery and those who encouraged me to have the new procedure. One specialist would not offer any advice without examining me and offered to do that right away. Two asked me to call them back, and two called me directly to give me advice over the phone. Some also offered to see me in their clinics within days. The difficulty in making the correct choice was apparent in some of the responses I received, as the responders outlined the strengths and weaknesses of each mode of surgery.

I was very grateful to all these otolaryngologists, some of whom I had never met before, for responding to my questions and for the useful information and offers to assist me in making the right choice. They truly came to my rescue at a most difficult time.

These were some of the responses I received:

"This is sad. You are one of my heroes. The older I get, the less I know. I am always worried about margins in this sort of cancer – which is prone to submucosal spread. As such, I would tend to want (if it were me) more extensive surgery – even if I ended up with a total laryngectomy. I am quite worried about aspiration in these sorts of cases – and, as much as I like to talk, I like to eat more. The risk of operating on someone famous is that we always tend to want to do a little less – and rely on hope."

"It must be a small recurrence that they think can be attempted this way. In the right hands, it has many advantages for recovery, but is not widely practiced (yet) – obviously cure is paramount, and after radiation this can be a difficult assessment (clear margins intra-operatively, etc). It may seem advantageous because one could always do the big surgery. I would feel more open to this approach before radiation, but now afterwards would be more inclined to salvage with an open procedure for cure. Hypopharynx cancers are usually difficult to cure long-term and both necks need to be done."

"Before I even read the endoscopic part, I began thinking, *Why don't they do an endoscopic resection?* The best case with endoscopic resection is that your tumor is gone, you function well, and you avoid a tracheotomy (possible). The lesser scenario involves another question: What you do if the margins were not clear or if your function was not good? In either case, you would require the 'bigger' surgery. You do not burn any bridges by having the endoscopic resection done as primary method. I know you will do well... I am happy to help in any other way."

"Both are options. Experience with laser resection is more limited. Without knowing all details and without my examination under anesthesia, it would be impossible for me to advise. The fact that it is PET-negative is puzzling and should be discussed with your surgeons."

"I am sorry to hear about your situation. Your question about the reliability of an endoscopic resection is difficult to answer because it is dependent upon a number of factors:

1) The extent of the tumor and depth of invasion. It may not be possible to completely determine these factors before trying to resection the tumor.
2) The experience of the surgeon in these procedures. Steiner in Germany is the most experienced with this technique. Drs. ..... and ..... at the University of ..... have been working on this extensively and probably have as much experience with this as anyone in the country. Unfortunately, no one has extensive experience.

In addition, some centers are re-irradiating after resection of these tumors. Depending on the size of the tumor and the margins, you might consider getting re-irradiation on a research protocol. This can improve your chances significantly.

You probably do not lose much by trying an endoscopic resection as long as you have close monitoring. Unfortunately, we generally have poor success with preserving the larynx in resections such as this. I would be prepared to possibly lose your larynx unless the tumor is very small."

"I am so sorry to hear about your dilemma. Resection of the pyriform with partial laryngectomy and reconstruction is not usually associated with very good functional outcome. Problems with aspiration are typical. Often, we will lean toward a total laryngopharyngectomy in these cases. I have limited experience with endoscopic resection in this area, but if the tumor has well-defined borders and a limited resection is feasible, then the functional outcomes are often better than with the more extensive surgery you describe. The fact that the two tumors are relatively close together implies that there are probably mucosal changes that extend broadly across the hypopharynx. This might make a limited resection unsatisfactory for complete tumor control. I would be happy to see you in the office to review things. Let me know if I can help."

"This can be a tough situation with hypopharyngeal carcinomas after radiation therapy, but laryngeal preservation can sometime be safely and functionally performed with transoral laser microsurgery. It depends on the location of the tumor and its extent. Hypopharyngeal cancers have a predilection for submucosal spread, so any conservative treatment should be very carefully considered. Let me know how I can help. I'd be happy to take a look at you in ..... on Monday."

"I am so sorry to hear of the recurrence that you have suffered. I have taken the liberty of talking to two of the head and neck oncologists that are in our department. Both are of the opinion that transoral laser resection would be the preferred next step. The technique allows for complete resection while minimizing the effects of the surgery. Please let me know if there is anything that I can do to help."

"I am reluctant to offer advice or comment on your specific case with the limited information one can get over an email. The decision to proceed with open or endoscopic resection depends on many factors, including the size and location of the tumor and the operator's experience and expertise. In general, salvage surgery after radiation needs to be extensive enough to have a hope of achieving clear margins."

"This is a really difficult question. There is growing literature reporting success with endoscopic piecemeal resection of hypopharyngeal cancer. Some have also undertaken these procedures for recurrent disease. In the end the real issue is: Can the whole tumor be removed? In the setting of prior radiation, this issue is especially difficult to answer. Is this truly a second primary – a reflection of multifocal disease or a submucosal metastasis? Under either circumstance, the potential for the presence of clinically undetectable disease outside the confines of the apparent tumor is high.

As I see it, there are three potential approaches: 1) a local resection, hoping this is the entire tumor; 2) a total laryngopharyngectomy with reconstruction, which offers the best potential for complete removal of multifocal disease, though it will not control distant metastasis and a free flap will be needed; and 3) re-irradiation with chemotherapy, for there is pretty good evidence that [it works in] about 30 percent, though this is associated with severe fibrosis and about 30 percent high-grade toxicity.

Option 1 sounds easiest but probably has the lowest potential for cure. Without a crystal ball, this is really difficult."

I shared some of these emails with my own surgeons, and this is the email response I received from one of them after he read the last message:

"I read Dr. ..... recommendations. The fact that you have a recurrence (be it a second primary, multifocal disease, or submucosal metastasis) does make local resection (endoscopic resection or partial pharyngectomy) less favorable. Of the three options he mentioned, total laryngopharyngectomy is probably the most aggressive, in that it removes all the mucosa at risk; however, it involves removing your larynx along with your hypopharynx and cancer. Chemo-radiation is another option, but is probably associated with the most toxicity. In some patients, the severe fibrosis as a late sequalae can result in marked dysphagia and aspiration, requiring a total laryngopharyngectomy with free flap reconstruction.

Thus, the local resection becomes, in my opinion, the best option. Keep in mind that when we go to the operating room, the goal is for total local resection of the tumor and a margin of normal tissue surrounding it. I don't suspect this will involve resecting any portion of the larynx but you need to understand that this is always a possibility. The plan is for direct laryngoscopy to reevaluate the tumor and to assess whether or not the tumor can be resectioned endoscopically. If not, we will convert to an open procedure (partial pharyngectomy with or without partial laryngectomy). Is this how you would like us to proceed?

I look forward to meeting you, your wife, and any other family members to discuss your case further and go over the risks and benefits of surgery."

The most informative email came among the last ones and was from Germany, from one of the most experienced surgeons in cancer laser surgery in the world. He also stressed the importance of experience in laser surgery:

"During the last two decades, we have expanded indications for laser surgery to almost all regions and tumor categories of the upper aero digestive tract. This even includes recurrent cancer, for which laser surgery also represents a valuable treatment option. However, especially after primary radiotherapy, surgeons have to be aware that recurrent tumors often grow diffusely within scarred tissue, which makes staging very difficult.

Many recurrent tumors are more advanced than they appear in diagnostic endoscopy and CT scan. It therefore requires much experience on part of the laser surgeon to recognize the true extension of the tumor and to remove it with histologically clear resection margins.

If you would be my patient and your tumor could be adequately exposed by endoscopy, I would clearly recommend transoral laser surgery (with neck dissection). The advantage of this approach is not only less morbidity than after conventional surgery (usually no tracheotomy!), but also the possibility to apply further surgical treatment from outside in case laser removal fails. All options are still maintained!! After surgery, I would recommend intensive follow-up, probably including two or three endoscopic investigations in full anesthesia during the first two years.

The main problem for you may be to find a laser surgeon who is experienced enough; especially in the treatment of recurrent tumors after radiotherapy (I do not know Dr.[Strom]). This would also be problematic in our country, as it is estimated that not more than five ear, nose, and throat departments in Germany are able to offer such high-end laser surgery that is necessary in your case."

The last message was from one of the laser experts surgeons in the USA:

"I think endoscopic laser resection is an excellent option for you if an experienced surgeon with this technique can expose it and resection it. The alternative is a fairly morbid operation, which you can always have if Transoral Laser Microsurgery fails (early or late). Our series on hypopharyngeal cancer treated with Transoral Laser Microsurgery is not yet in print (in press now) but is encouraging when compared to standard therapy. It's all about exposure and resectability. I would encourage you to let them try the endoscopic approach up front. You really have nothing to lose and might get a nice result without the long hospital stay, tracheotomy, and donor site morbidity of the flap. Let me know if I can help in any way, and good luck. Sorry you have to go through this."

Dr. Ross, another laser surgeon from the USA was very helpful to me and described to me over the phone the details of his therapeutic approach. He was also willing to see me and operate on me after an initial evaluation. I was tempted to travel to his center but realized that this would further delay the removal of my tumor. However, I informed my surgeons about his advice and methodology and asked them to contact him so that they could benefit from his experience:

"I have just talked with Dr. [Ross] from the University of ... who does about 120 cases a year of transoral laser resection, including those of the pyriform sinus area. He believes that this can be an adequate approach in my case but talked to me at length about the importance of adequate margins, especially in recurrence or secondary primary. He told me that prior to surgery, he does mucosal mapping with several biopsies of the entire area, including the original primary site to make sure that there is no microscopic recurrence. He also told me that after resecting the tumor, he ensures that the margins around it are clear at all directions and also deep under the resected area. Sometimes the frozen section is negative, but later in definite microscopy they find them to be positive. They then would go back and complete the resection.

I was very impressed by Dr. [Ross's] knowledge and careful approach. He said that he would be very happy to discuss this with you. I would very much appreciate if you would. His phone number is enclosed. Thanks again for everything."

I have no idea if my surgeons called that expert in laser surgery who offered to help. However, Dr. Strom responded to my sharing with him all the messages I had received:

"I sincerely appreciate the information/contacts you have provided. I feel confident that an initial endoscopic approach is reasonable in your case. We will, of course, take multiple mapping biopsies, from both your new primary site and old site. If it appears that there is widespread submucosal involvement, we will stop at that point, wake you up, and discuss the options. Reason being, if you have extensive submucosal disease, you may need a significant resection with high morbidity. There could be the possibility of primary chemotherapy at this point with surgical salvage. We can discuss this more tomorrow."

The overall impression I got from all these communications was that my surgeons' approach was reasonable and that I should proceed to undergo laser surgery. Although I had the option of traveling to a different medical center to undergo that operation, I elected to let the local specialists do it. While some of the communications I received warned me that the success of this approach depended on the operator's experience, I was not too concerned with my surgeons' expertise.

As part of the preparation for the upcoming surgery, I was examined by a dentist and SLPs. Prior to this, I had had very minimal contact or experience with SLPs and did not realize what a pivotal role they play in the recovery and life after laryngectomy. I was to see the SLP in case I had a total laryngectomy and lost my vocal cords. The SLP explained to me why my ability to speak would not go away if this happened and elaborated about the three potential methods by which I could vocalize. I learned that all that the vocal cords do is generate vibration and the actual formation of words is done by the tongue and lips. Such vibration can be generated either by air that is "burped" out from the stomach (in esophageal speech), by an external artificial larynx (an Electro-Larynx) placed on the cheeks or under the chin, or by a tracheo-esophageal prosthesis that would connect my trachea and esophagus using a small hole that would be created during my surgery (TEP).

The information I received was reassuring because I better understood the speech alternatives to vocal cords. However, I did not think that I would ever need to use any of these options, and deep inside I believed that I would never loss my natural voice.

When I met with Dr. Cooper for the last time prior to surgery, I decided to ask him about his experience using laser to remove my type of cancer. I had never challenged a physician directly before, questioning their expertise. I felt apprehensive in doing that, as it might have manifested a lack of trust but since the stakes were so high, I decided to ask.

He openly and honestly told me that although he had used laser on numerous occasions, he had operated only once on a case such as myself. "How did the patient do after surgery?" I asked.

"The surgery went well," he replied, "but the patient died later because his cancer had spread to his lungs." I asked him again how confident is he about using laser on me, to which he responded while looking straight into my eyes, "If I felt that I could not do it, I would tell you so. I am confident I can do it well." His confidence and reassurance made me feel very comfortable in him and his team. He also assured me that he was going to use the best and most sophisticated laser instrument, similar to the one used by the most experienced medical centers who perform such surgeries in Germany.

All was set for the big day. I felt that I had covered all ground and chosen the best option for myself. What was left was just a little more waiting time.

Six days prior to the surgery, I gave a lecture to an intensive care unit staff at one of the hospitals in my area. I was very much aware that the lecture may have been my last using my normal voice. I did not share my impending operation with any of the listeners. However, when I was offered the gift of a board that contained essential communication words and signs that could be used by patients who are unable to speak, I took it with me. These fundamental words illustrated how helpless one can be after laryngectomy, including things like "I have pain... Suction me... Yes... No... Water." As reluctant as I was to take such a gift, it unfortunately proved very useful in the weeks that followed.

Chapter 9. Did Laser Surgery Work?

One month after the recurrent cancer was diagnosed, I arrived at the Army Hospital at four forty-five a.m. on a cold January morning. My wife, son, and my oldest daughter (whose wedding we had attended twenty-one months ago) came all the way from California to accompany me. I tried to dissuade my daughter from taking the long trip, mainly because she had endured several miscarriages, but she insisted on coming. My middle daughter was planning to arrive later that day and see me after the surgery.

When we arrived, the surgical waiting room was already full of patients and their family members, and we barely found room to sit down. I was issued a bracelet that I had to wear on my wrist which bore my name, and I was given a hospital gown to replace my street clothes. The bracelet was very loosely fitted and kept falling down. There were papers I had to sign in addition to the ones I had already signed about a week earlier at the pre-surgical examinations I had taken.

What followed was a long wait. Even though I was worried and nervous, I did my best to conceal those feelings. *Why were we told to come so early if we have to wait so long?* I wondered. It was interesting to watch the faces of the other patients and their family members. There was a strange silence in the room – some kind of tense expectation and fear of the unknown. Some patients were waiting for simple procedures, but others (like me) were facing long, complicated surgeries where the outcome and risks were much greater.

At about six a.m., we were all asked to get up and line up in the corridor outside the waiting room. After we formed a long row of about twenty patients and a greater number of family members and friends, we were marched down the hospital corridors to the elevators that took us to the operating room floor, where we were asked to form the long column again and march to our destination.

This method of taking the patients to the operating room was very strange and impersonal, funny in a way but also seriously wrong. The formation was similar to the one used in military marches and was definitely inappropriate in that setting. It was similar to the way I was instructed to march in formation as a regular enlisted soldier many years ago in Israel. Even though this was a military hospital, most of the patients were elderly and were either retirees or non-military dependents, as were most of their family members. Interestingly, though, none of the hospital personnel who organized the march were active members of the military. It was disconcerting to see the long row of patients wearing hospital clothes being led in such a blatantly impersonal way to a place were they were going to undergo major surgery. Some patients would come out of the procedures they were about to have substantially changed, and a few might even not make it through. The march of patients down the halls was ominously reminiscent of prisoners being led to the gallows.

The impersonal march increased the worry and anxiety that I was experiencing prior to the surgery. *Is this the way to treat people who are hungry, tense, worried, and afraid of the unknown?* I had surgeries before at other military and non-military hospitals and had never experienced such a dehumanizing experience. I had always appreciated the personal attention and individual care that I had received at other hospitals, which made it easier to face the impending surgery.

We were then told to line up opposite the wall at the entrance of the operating room, and the staff began calling up individual patients and directing them to their beds at the preparatory areas. At that stage, we were told that our family members could no longer accompany us. I said goodbye to my family, asked them not to worry, and reminded them to go to the waiting room where the surgeons would update them about the progress of my operation.

The next phase was more pleasant and personal, as I had my vital signs taken, an intravenous infusion started, and I met the anesthetist and his nurse. I was reassured by their kindness and self-confidence and felt they were there to do their best for me. I was then wheeled down to the operating room.

I was surprised to find the large operating room to be very crowded. I counted at least twenty-two individuals and observed several large pieces of equipment that filled the room up beyond its capacity. In addition to the surgical trays and anesthesia machines, I observed a microscope for the pathologist and a sophisticated laser apparatus that had numerous adjacent gadgets. In addition to the four surgeons, there were several nurses, two anesthetists, and a technician from the manufacturer of the laser machine equipment, who I later learned had lent that apparatus to my surgeon especially for this surgery. In retrospect, the fact that this was the first time my surgeons had used that laser instrument was disconcerting, and I wished that they would have had more experience in using it. The room was so crowded that I could not be wheeled to the operating table. I volunteered to get off of my gurney and walked over and between the multiple pieces of equipment to the operating table, where I lay down. The orderly was surprised at my move, but it made me feel good that I could solve the problem quickly and walk into the operating room not as a helpless patient. I knew I would not be able to exit that way.

Once I entered the operating room, my anxiety and apprehension subsided to a large extent, and I felt an inner strength and resolve that boosted my spirits. I was determined to go through the ordeal I was facing. I was also amazed and heartened by the large number of people who gathered in the operating room to take care of me. It made me feel more confident that things would turn out all right if so much talent and experience were gathered in one room. I had not previously known that what I was to undergo required so much manpower and effort. I felt great gratitude to all of the medical personal gathered in the operating room, and just before going under the anesthesia, I thanked everyone for what they were going to do for me and wished them good luck.

I woke up several hours later and found myself in the SICU breathing through an oxygen mask and connected to intravenous and arterial lines, as well as monitoring instruments. I also had a urine catheter and a tube which was placed in my nose for feeding and delivery of liquids, including oral medications. I was elated to realize that I could speak and did not have to breathe through a tracheostomy tube. This meant that I had been spared from losing my vocal cords. My recollection of the events during the early hours after my surgery is vague, but it improved slowly with time. However, because I was receiving narcotics and other medications, whatever I remember is very fuzzy. Even though I was offered to self-administer my narcotics through an automated intravenous pump, I refused to do that and asked the nurses not to give me those medications so that I could be more alert and return to my senses. I did it mostly because I felt that my pain was tolerable and could be treated without narcotic painkillers that have significant side effects. I also wanted to be able to monitor my condition myself, and becoming sleepier would interfere with this. I requested only Tylenol for the pain, and that seemed to be enough.

I learned later that my family members had visited me for a short time soon after I was brought to the SICU, but they were not allowed to stay for long. I also heard from them that the surgeons updated them about their initial findings, as well as the progress of my operation which lasted about seven hours.

I had one-on-one care by nurses throughout my stay in the SICU, and they were very competent and efficient and performed all the necessary procedures. These included suctioning, monitoring my vital signs, and administration of medication. As I slowly came back to my senses, I realized that, as expected, I had a large bandage covering the right side of my neck, and my throat was very painful. I had no sensation on the right side of my neck because the lymph glands there were removed in case the cancer had spread. During the process of removing these glands, the nerves at that area were cut off. Unfortunately, the sensation deficit was permanent.

I also felt that I was missing one of my right lower molars. I remember being told by Dr. Cooper that a tooth was inadvertently broken off by him when he manipulated the endoscope used to remove the tumor. He had not realized it broke off until he found the tooth lodged in my trachea.

The surgeons were very happy to inform me that my surgery was a great success. It went very well and was executed as planned. They were able to remove the cancer in its entirety by using the laser, and all the margins of the removed area were clear of cancer. I was therefore spared from the more extensive surgery, which would have included removal of tissues in the right side of my neck, requiring their replacement by tissues transplanted from my thighs or shoulder areas. However, as was planned, the entire lymph gland system in the right side of my neck was excised and was going to be studied for the presence of metastasis within a few days.

Despite my hazy state of mind, I felt great relief when I heard the news and felt very fortunate. Even though there was still uncertainty about the final pathological results, the alternative was much worse.

The night that followed was a long one, and I did not get much sleep in the noisy SICU. Surprisingly, I did not feel too tired. The SICU physicians and my surgeons assured me on their morning rounds that I was doing quite well, and the plan was to continue the present treatment and monitor my progress. They attempted to lower my blood pressure which became elevated following the surgery because of the large amounts of fluids I had received during the procedure.

One of the annoying problems I experienced was that I could not swallow my saliva without having pain in my throat. I solved that problem during my awake hours by repeatedly suctioning my mouth with a catheter. However, I could not do that while I was sleeping, and the painful swallowing kept me from falling asleep. I finally found a position where I could sit up and lean forward to allow the secretion to run into a towel. However, this did not work so well. Finally, with the help of a nurse, I was able to put my head down in a sitting position on several pillows which allowed me some badly needed time to sleep. This problem haunted me throughout my hospitalization, but fortunately it abated in its intensity over time.

The second night in the SICU was again a sleepless one. In the morning, my arterial line and urine catheter were removed, and I was relieved to be able to pass urine myself. Since I was doing so well in my recovery, I was to be moved to the regular surgical unit later that day.

When I was finally moved out of the SICU, I appreciated how large and crowded the place was, which I was unable to note from my separate cubicle. I was looking forward to leaving the SICU and going to the regular ward. It meant to me that I was on the right course of recovery that would lead to my ultimate discharge from the hospital. It would also allow me to finally see and spend more time with my family and friends. Unfortunately, what was waiting for me was an unnerving and frustrating hospitalization where I encountered numerous problems and deficiencies in my nursing care. It was very surprising for me to discover these problems. Even though I had served as a consultant and an attending physician in that hospital for many years, I had never appreciated how common these mistakes were. It was different to experience that place as a patient.

Because of a shortage in nurses, many of the nursing positions in military hospitals (especially the Army ones) are staffed by civilian nurses. I found that, in general, I could expect better care from military staff personnel as compared to civilian nurses. Military personnel and nurses had more uniform training, were more disciplined and followed the nursing role more closely than their civilian counterparts.

I was admitted to a two-patient room in the regular surgical ward. I shared the room with a patient who had had numerous orthopedic surgeries in his leg after being wounded during the Iraq war. I was moved after a few hours to a smaller single-patient room on the same floor that had become vacant, which made it easier for me and my family.

The first upsetting event occurred after I had been in the ward for less than an hour. I had requested my surgeons to get an urgent dental consult for me. I was concerned about my broken tooth and wanted to be seen by a dentist as soon as possible. Not only did the sharp edges of the fractured tooth irritate my tongue, but I was also concerned that if it were not sealed immediately, it would become infected and subsequently lost. This was of greater concern in my case since I had received irradiation to that area. The irradiation to the neck often compromises the blood supply to the lower jaw, which would have required administration of hyperbaric oxygen prior to any extensive dental work at that area.

I was very glad to be visited at my bedside by a dentist minutes after arriving on the floor. After briefly inspecting my tooth and realizing the potential complexity of my situation, she told me that she would return in a short while with her attending. She came back escorted by her uniformed senior staff dentist, Dr. Ken, who also inspected my mouth. He was very short-tempered and treated me abruptly and impersonally almost to the point of rudeness, ignoring my questions and input. When he concluded his examination, he initiated a discussion with the younger dentist about his treatment plan, which was to seal the broken tooth until it could be reconstructed.

Dr. Ken seemed to be very knowledgeable in the methods and precautions required when treating someone after irradiation. When he finished his analysis, I voiced my agreement with his treatment plan by simply saying, "I agree."

He reacted to my remark by snapping at me with an angry outburst. "If you know so much about dental care, why did you ask me to come and see you?!" This was done in a contemptuous manner and to hear it from a senior military officer made it even more insulting. I was not only hurt to be treated like this by a medical colleague, but also felt humiliated as an ordinary patient. *How can a health professional be so insensitive to a patient that has just undergone a major surgical procedure and is under his care?* The incident happened in a crowded hospital room and was witnessed by my family and the other patient and his guests.

In retrospect, I assume that the dentist had no idea that I was a physician and was unaware of my extensive knowledge in dentistry and oral pathology. Not only did I have experience in complex dental procedures (because I had numerous dental problems in the past), but much of my research and writings were on dental topics. It was natural for me to listen to his deliberations and voice my support because his reasoning was very sound. However, even if I had none of these qualifications, there was no reason to be treated in such a contemptuous manner.

I felt so upset about it that I could not hold back a reaction to his insult. The high rank of the dentist did not intimidate me as it might have if I have been still on active duty. I also noticed even before this occurrence that, after I was diagnosed with cancer, I became less inhibited in speaking out whenever I felt insulted. Even though I was still very weak and my voice was not strong, I told the dentist how rude he was and how unprofessional his attitude and response to me was. My oldest daughter joined me to further reiterate how inappropriate he was. Her support at that time as my advocate was very helpful and brought home the message.

I could see that the dentist was taken aback by our response. He probably was not used to hearing patients (or anyone else) talk back to him, telling him the truth straight in his face. He did not apologize but obviously got the message that we were not planning to stop there and, if needed, we were going to pursue this matter further up the chain of command to the hospital administration. Dr. Ken told me that he was going to take care of me right away and personally wheeled me to his clinic where one of his residents took care of the tooth by temporarily sealing it and smoothing it out. He was vague about whether he planned to have it fixed later, but I never came back to his clinic and got the tooth permanently repaired at the Navy Dental clinic instead.

This incident left a very bitter taste. The insult, humiliation, and anger stayed for a while. I wondered if other patients had also suffered similar insults from that dentist. I never pursued a formal complaint about this incident, for I was struggling with too many other important issues relating to my recovery. When I conveyed this experience to my surgeon, he shared my frustration but did not do anything about it.

Unfortunately, this incident was just the beginning of a series of others, albeit more incompetence than rudeness. In addition to those discussed here, there were many other minor problems. I was able to observe and correct some only after I felt stronger. Fortunately, I was surrounded by family members who observed many errors themselves and helped me assure that they were not repeated. I was wondering how many mistakes are made in good and reputable medical institutions that are unnoticed by patients and family members without medical background. Realizing that I had to be my own watchman consumed much of my energy at a time when I needed all of my strength to recuperate.

My oldest daughter became my main advocate in watching over me and assuring everything was done right. She was not bashful about voicing her concerns and following them up all the way to the supervisors. I was often the one who noticed the infraction and told her about it, but she often picked up on them herself. However, once we realized that there were so many things going wrong, she often overdid it, even when it was not necessary. One of my concerns about being too vigilant was that it might create animosity toward me by the personnel I depended on for essential support and care.

Hospitals can be very dangerous places for patients, and it is a miracle that most leave without any permanent damage inadvertently inflicted on them by well-intentioned staff members who are negligent, overworked or poorly trained. This was a shocking realization for me, even though I had spent my entire medical career in these settings. As a patient, I gained a new perspective.

Within my first twenty-four hours at the surgical ward, these errors became very obvious. When I was admitted around noon to the regular ward, the licensed practical nurses (LPN) who checked me did not perform a full physical assessment including examination of the heart and lungs using a stethoscope. A complete physical examination was performed only after my family requested that a registered nurse (RN) take care of me after the LPN suggested that my family request RN care. This was delayed until a nightshift switch took place.

Even though my tube feeding was ordered early in the day, it was not started until late in the evening because the staff was too busy. The LPN claimed that she had to check with a RN for orders, which delayed the process and my care. I experienced several choking episodes during that evening because the feeding was done in a faster than usual rate in an attempt to deliver the necessary daily amount of feeding.

Even though I was not to receive anything by mouth, when my medicines were to be given that evening the RN came into my room and suggested I take them by mouth with a cup and water and said it was OK to use ice chips. When she was told by my daughter that I was not to receive anything orally, she admitted that she had not read the doctor's orders.

Since I developed a headache my doctors ordered Tylenol. My orders for the liquid medicine were for adult dosage; however, the RN wanted to administer a pediatric dosage. I had to inform her myself that these dosages were for pediatric patients and would be ineffective. Subsequently, she had to page the doctor on call and get new orders.

I experienced intense episodes of persistent migraine headaches for which Imitrix (either twenty-five mg. in liquid or its equivalent amount in injection, which was only six mg.) was prescribed by the doctor. The RN wanted to inject me with four ampoules of six -mg. Imitrex each to get equivalence to the oral dose. I stopped her from doing that because this would have been an inappropriately high dose with dangerous cardiac toxicity that could have been deadly. She was obviously unfamiliar with the injection dose and had communication problems with both the doctor on call and the pharmacy. This caused a delay of several hours, with my pain becoming unbearable. Even though I repeatedly told the nurse that six-mg. Imitrix injection was equivalent to twenty-five mg. oral Imitrix no one seemed to know that.

When attempting to deliver my medications, a nurse inserted a syringe into my feeding tube forcefully without removing its cap. I had to stop her from damaging the tube and educate her about the need to remove the cover before using the syringe. The feeding tube could have been damaged because of the forceful and inappropriate insertion.

Because my electrical hospital bed was constantly generating mechanical noise, I requested the nurse to unplug it. My family noticed a few hours later that he had also unplugged the intravenous pump, which subsequently ceased deliver intravenous fluids to me after the battery was exhausted.

On the second day, I experienced difficulty in swallowing and had repeated choking episodes because dry mucous got stuck in my airways and throat. I asked the nurse for humidified air to prevent the mucus from becoming dry. She told me that this would require a Respiratory Services consultation. I was under the assumption that the nurse had requested that the doctors ask for the consultation, but I learned later she did not. Even after the doctors ordered a face mask for humidification, it was not delivered for many hours. I was told hours later that it was not available. With no help available, my family had to bring in a day later a humidifier from our home that I used throughout my hospitalization.

After orders were placed to remove one of the two intravenous lines, a nurse came in to do it and asked me which of the lines had to be removed. Was it my role to know?

These repeated nursing errors were so unnerving and upsetting that my family and I conveyed them to the doctors and nursing supervisor. The nursing supervisor was very attentive and promised to look into these problems and asked my family to write them down. We also had a visitor from the hospital public relations department, who listened to my family's complaints and promised to help. They were very dismayed and apologetic and, in an attempt to mend the situation came back and informed me that I was going to be moved to another ward in the hospital – a ward that served only very important persons (VIPs) and dignitaries. The ward had only eight beds and was securely placed behind locked double doors at the upper floor of the hospital.

I had never heard about that ward before because its existence was kept quiet for security and public relations reasons. I learned later that its presence drew media scrutiny, especially because it showed that special preferential hospitalization conditions are given to select individuals while soldiers who risked their lives in battle are treated in crowded wards.

The offer to be moved away from the surgical ward came to me as a surprise. I did not object to the move, but I had no idea where I was going to be taken. I was wheeled away to the hospital top floor through a side corridor and security locked double doors. Behind those doors was a beautifully decorated ward that looked more like a combination of a historical mansion and an expensive five-star hotel. The walls had pictures of President Eisenhower (the floor was named after him) and his wife, as well as other dignitaries. It was filled with antique style furniture, had an elegant dining and reception rooms, a library decorated with wall paintings and statues, and the corridors were filled with gifts given to the ward by world-famous dignitaries who had stayed on that floor. It also had a state-of-the-art conference room with sophisticated electronic equipment that could be used for worldwide conferencing and communication. The presents and guestbook revealed the names of some of these VIPs, including the Dali Lama, heads of states, world leaders, senators, retired generals, and diplomats.

My large room looked like an elegant hotel suite and was beautifully decorated and furnished. The only odd piece of furniture in the room was the hospital bed, but even it looked more like a hotel bed. The room had an elegant dining table, couches, sofas, and immaculate dressing and bathroom areas.

The floor had its own kitchen and a cook who wore a white chef hat. I was told that my own meal, as well those for my guests, could be ordered and cooked to our specifications, and an elaborate menu was given to us. I could not enjoy any of these special services, as I was still fed by a gastric tube; however, it was nice to offer my family tea in the afternoon.

The floor was staffed by an RN and a military corpsman, and since there were only two more patients in that ward, I had very personal and immediate attention, and the care I received was immaculate.

However, since the floor was not a surgical floor and was used more often for medical treatment, the nurses there were less familiar with post-surgical care and had some trouble changing my dressings and manipulating the suction equipment.

One of the happiest events that occurred during my stay on that floor was to hear that my oldest daughter had learned she was pregnant. This was a very happy occasion for all of us, because she had been trying to become pregnant for a long time.

Since my doctors encouraged me to take short strolls, I walked up and down the beautiful but empty corridors, stopping and inspecting the statues, paintings, the gifts and their inscriptions and read the guestbook, enjoying what had been written by all the famous people. The place was very quiet, and I felt strangely out of place – like a visitor to a national museum. However, it was not hard for me to get used to the elegant surroundings.

I was very grateful to have been moved to this tranquil and beautiful place. I was hoping that this move also illustrated the hospital's gratitude to me for my long service to the medical community, including that facility, as well to the military at large. I thought I was moved to the ward because I was important enough in their eyes that they honored me by having me stay where VIPs from this country and the world stayed.

However, my stay at this location was quite short. Less than two days after my transfer, I was told by the RN that I was to be moved back to the surgical floor. The explanation was that the VIP floor was soon to become crowded by newly-admitted VIPs, and since they did not have enough staff to handle too many patients, I had to leave. I was upset and felt insulted and humiliated by the sudden news. I had mistakenly thought I would complete my hospital stay at that location and would not be moved again. All the thoughts that the transfer was the result of gratitude evaporated. In retrospect, I wish I would have not been taken to that floor in the first place so that I would not have experienced the letdown and rejection caused by vacating the ward.

Before I left the ward, I added my name to the guestbook, as was done by previous patients. I used a page to thank the staff and doctors for their care. I signed my name in both English and Hebrew and wrote down my military ranks at both the US Navy and Israeli military. I thought this would be a nice way to summarize my past military services.

I was afraid that I would face errors and nursing problems again when I returned to the regular floor. However, my doctors assured me that my stay would be better because they were going to transfer me to a different ward that had the reputation of being better and more efficient. One of my surgeons shared with me how uncomfortable he felt about having a floor such as the VIP floor. He believed that there should not be any class distinctions in medical care delivery in the military, and, in his opinion, generals and politicians should be treated in the same facilities used to treat ordinary line soldiers and their dependants. In retrospect, I fully agree with him, although at that time I still felt the insult of being "demoted" back to a regular ward.

I was moved to a single-patient room in a different ward and was hoping to have a better experience this time. However, even though the care was generally more attentive on the new ward, there were again multiple errors and incidents of inappropriate care.

A short time after my transfer, the charge nurse gave me a brief physical examination. Learning from our previous experiences, my family requested that I receive care from an RN and not LPN. However, even though I was admitted to the floor at one p.m., no nurse came into my room until eight-thirty p.m. When no medicines were given to me at the scheduled time of six p.m., my family members reminded the nurses about it and were told that these medications had not yet been delivered to the floor. Apparently, the pharmacy was not informed about my transfer, so my medications were erroneously still being sent up to the VIP floor. My daughter had to go to the former floor to ask them to ship the medications to the new location. Since no nurse came to my room after repeated requests, I had to insert water into my feeding tube myself. I finally received the six p.m. medicines at eight-thirty p.m. The tube feeding that was supposed to start at seven p.m. did not begin until nine-fifteen p.m.

At ten p.m., a nurse came to give me oral antibiotics through the oral tube. Instead of bringing a suspension of the drug, she crushed down pills in water. The pills were not adequately crushed and kept clogging the feeding tube. When I asked her to crush the pills again, she suggested that I swallow them, not understanding that I was not to receive anything by mouth because the surgical area in my throat was to be spared from any contact with food or other substances. I was wondering how an RN could be unaware of patient condition to that extreme.

The next morning, an RN came to inspect my surgical wounds, which, to my surprise, she planned to do without sterile gloves. I politely reminded her to wear them. Because my identification bracelet was very loose and kept easily slipping off, I requested she replace it. However, no new bracelet was delivered for several days, during which I had to keep reminding the nurses about it. Having the patient wear an identity bracelet at all times is essential in preventing medical errors.

A nursing assistant took my blood pressure using an inappropriately large blood pressure cuff. Using too large a cuff produces erroneous blood pressure measurement lower than the true one. Indeed, the blood pressure she got was 124/78, which is normal. I told her that she needed to use a cuff that covered about two-thirds of my arm. Arguing with me, she asked me if the blood pressure she took is my regular blood pressure. I explained to her that there is no predicated regular blood pressure in a patient and that this has to be measured to determine it. I had to ask her to use an appropriate cuff size (in proportion to my arm) to obtain an accurate reading. When she reluctantly did so, she obtained a reading of 149/86, which was clinically elevated. This is an example of how using an inappropriate method leads to documentation of an incorrect measurement. In my case, reporting a "normal" finding would have prevented the doctors from intervening to lower my elevated blood pressure. I wondered how often such mistakes lead to serious consequences. As a physician, I was able to avert that error, but what could a lay person do – just suffer the consequences?

On the second day in the ward, a nurse came into my room and informed me that I had a dentist appointment in the dental clinic. After I told her that I was not aware of such an appointment, she asked a student nurse to call the clinic. The clinic told her that I had no appointment scheduled. Apparently, she did not convey that information to the nurse who came back into my room and told me that a dentist was waiting for me in the dental clinic. I asked her for the name of the dentist, but she did not know. Instead, she insisted that I needed to be taken to the clinic without delay.

When I arrived at the dental clinic, I was told to stay in the waiting room. I got no answer to my question about which dentist it was who would see me. I did not protest when I was taken to have several X-rays of my mouth. I thought they were ordered by my expectant dentist. I was sent back to the patient waiting area and still had no idea who was going to see me. After one hour of investigation and talking to the resident dentist who saw me five days earlier, I was told that I had no dental appointment. No one in the clinic or the ward could give me a logical explanation for what had occurred and why I had been exposed to unnecessary X-rays. The only explanation I received was that the error "most probably occurred" because another patient with a similar name and number had an appointment that day. Because of the time I wasted at the dental clinic, my medicine administration was delayed by an hour.

Post-surgical stay is not easy. Being nourished by intravenous fluids and feeding tube is difficult and annoying. The feeding tube that was inserted into my nose started to hurt and caused local redness and inflammation after a few days. My surgeons removed it once and placed a new one in the other nostril, but this also caused me local irritation. I felt great relief when my surgeons finally removed my feeding tube and allowed me to receive liquids by mouth. As I was getting physically stronger, I was looking forward to leaving the hospital, especially because I realized that it was not the safest place to be.

Even though I no longer required intravenous fluids, I had to have an intravenous access line through a needle that was stuck in the back of my palm. Such a line was placed in all hospitalized patients and was to be used in case of a medical emergency. To maintain the patency of the line, it had to be flushed with saline every twelve hours and changed at least every seventy-two hours. To avoid clogging the line and insertion of a new needle, I tried to do my best to protect the needle site. However, after a day or so, the injection site started to be irritating and painful. It was a relief to finally get the needle out before my discharge.

My family members were with me at almost all times, especially on the first days of my hospital stay. They made sure that someone was always there to stay overnight and watch over me. This was actually very helpful on the first night of my stay in the regular ward where I had several bouts of choking caused by coughing up thick mucus and required suctioning of my airways. When the nurses failed to come to my assistance, my daughter rushed to the nurses' station and got their help. My family's presence was very comforting, and they assisted me in the various chores and tasks I had to perform.

They were very vigilant and made sure that I get the proper attention from the nursing staff, especially during the first five post-surgical days when I was bedridden. I had to remind them on many occasions to let me use the CALL button to get help because they had become used to walking to the nurses' station directly to seek assistance. However, once I started to feel better, I preferred to be left alone at night because the presence of one of my children in the room made me refrain from coughing or calling for assistance; I did not want to wake them up.

On numerous occasions, especially during the first post-surgical days when I was still weak and very tired, my family members were the ones who observed most of the errors and infractions in my care and made sure they were corrected.

I felt bad about the toll and burden that the constant hospital stay imposed on my family members and tried to dissuade them from spending so many hours there. I had to request and insist that they go home every night. In the first days of my hospitalization, I did it because I wanted them to get some respite from the constant burden of caring for me. However, as I became stronger, I did it also because I needed time alone and actually could relax and rest much better when I was by myself. I realized then that the constant presence of guests and family members is quite taxing and can be tiring. I encouraged them to take shifts and share the stay with each other so that they could have time to do other things. I told my middle and younger daughters that they could return to New York because my middle daughter had to take care of her five-year-old child and my youngest daughter had to teach her kindergarten class.

The day of my discharge finally arrived a week after my surgery. I was excited and happy to finally go home. Even though I had a turbulent and unsatisfactory post-surgical stay, I felt very fortunate to be cured from my cancer and not to have gone through a more extensive surgery. I kept asking my surgeons about the final pathological results, but they assured me that they would be soon available. Everything was looking great, and I was expecting to hear from them about the final report before going home.

The last day was dragging on and on, and my discharge orders were not in yet. I was not too concerned about the delay because I assumed this was due to my surgeons' busy schedule and that they would eventually get around to discharging me. Unfortunately, what was waiting for me dwarfed all the other problems and errors I had previously experienced.

Chapter 10. Chasing the Cancer

About four-thirty p.m., the chief otolaryngology resident, accompanied by a junior resident, walked into my room and asked me to follow them to the Otolaryngology Clinic. I was a little surprised because all I expected to receive from them were my discharge papers. They explained to me that they want to reexamine my upper airways one more time using endoscopy. This made sense and seemed reasonable to me because I assumed that they wanted to perform a final examination prior to my discharge. I expected this would take only a few minutes, and I would be allowed to finally go home.

In the clinic, they directed me to an examination room. I sat on the examination chair, and the senior resident numbed my upper airway and inserted the endoscope downward through my nose. He seemed to concentrate on one area and asked the junior resident to also observe it. They mumbled something incoherent to each other and nodded their heads in agreement. I asked them if everything was okay, but they did not respond. After completing their examination, they left my room without saying a word and closed the door. It felt strange to me to sit on the examination chair waiting for their return, but no one came back for a long time.

After sitting there for about thirty minutes, I left the examination room and searched the clinic to no avail, finding no one. I did not want to leave the clinic because I was expecting the doctors to come back any minute. I was concerned that my family members were worried about my whereabouts because they were not in my room when

I left. I called the ward and left a message to inform my family that I was in the clinic. The long wait was very unnerving and did not make any sense to me. However, I really had no suspicion that there was anything wrong.

After about fifty minutes, the two residents, accompanied by the two senior surgeons who performed my surgery, Drs. Strom and Cooper, walked into the room and delivered to me the most distressing and upsetting news.

Dr. Cooper began, "I would like to discuss with you the results of the pathological examinations. I have some good and some bad news. The good news is that there are no signs of cancer spreading into the lymph glands on the left side of the neck. The bad news is that the tumor is still in your hypopharynx. We have not yet removed it. The endoscopic examination done today confirmed that it is still where it was before."

Words cannot express the extent of my feelings when I heard the news. I was stunned. *How can this be possible? The surgeons didn't remove the whole tumor last week?* They had assured me they did, and the margins that were left around it were all negative. My first response was utter surprise and disbelief. Anger and loss of trust came later. Accepting my situation and making decisions for the best course of action came last.

The surgeon proceeded to explain that the tissue they removed with the endoscope was not the tumor, but rather scar tissue that looked abnormal. That abnormal area was only half an inch away from the cancer, but was higher up in my airway, so that when they inserted the endoscope, they observed it right away. Because that area looked very suspicious, they assumed that this was the tumor. They removed it and sent it to the pathological laboratory without confirming that what they took out was indeed cancerous. They then proceeded to take biopsies around the resected area. These biopsies were immediately frozen and inspected in the operating room and were found to be cancer-free. When the pathology laboratory read the resected tissue suspected to be cancerous several days later, to the surprise of everyone, there were no cancer cells to be seen, and the tissue contained only scar tissue. To my question why they did not do perform frozen sections of the tissue suspected to be cancerous in the operating room, Dr. Copper responded "We were convinced that what he had removed was the cancer."

Obviously, the surgeons erroneously assumed that they had removed the cancer. However, if they would have requested that the pathologist who was present in the operating room confirm this by looking at the frozen sections of the suspected cancerous lesion, the error would have been discovered right away and they would have proceeded to search and ultimately remove the cancer, which was so close by.

It was no surprise that the biopsies around the scar tissues were all negative. The surgeons discovered their mistake only when the pathological report came back and showed only scar tissue in the specimen. What was left now to do was to go back and attempt to remove the actual tumor. The surgeons informed me that they were planning to do just that in two days.

I was puzzled and upset by the incompetence of the surgeons. I had so many disturbing questions for them: "Why is this not the standard of care to immediately study by frozen section the removed tumor right in the operating room? This could have prevented me from needing another surgical procedure. Furthermore, this failure has delayed the removal of the cancer for nine additional days. How could you have missed finding the tumor you observed several times before?"

What was even more upsetting was that a few days prior to the surgery, my surgeon reassured me that he was going to take biopsies of the cancer before removing it and confirm the presence of cancer at the site. His email just prior to my surgery said, "I feel confident that an initial endoscopic approach is reasonable in your case. We will, of course, take multiple mapping biopsies, from both your new primary site and old site."

Later, I learned from the otolaryngologist that another adverse consequence of the failure to remove the cancer on the first surgery was that each surgery induces extensive local swelling and inflammation, rendering immediate surgery in the affected area more difficult. This was especially significant in my case because my tumor was located at a very narrow and difficult to access and visualize area. In other words, the best chance for successfully removal of the cancer by laser had been in the first surgery. After the initial surgery, the narrow passage where the tumor was situated became inflamed, irritated and swollen, and its diameter was therefore reduced. This made any follow-up interventions more difficult because insertion of an endoscope and visualization of the area were harder.

It was very difficult for me to contain my feelings of extreme anger and my loss of trust; but I knew it was inappropriate for me to express these emotions freely and in a non-inhibited way as I wished I could. I was very vulnerable and depended on these surgeons who were still taking care of me. I had close professional relationships with many of them for over twenty-seven years and liked them very much as individuals. I only wished I could tell them how angry I was and walk away to get treatment elsewhere. I regretted not having the laser surgery done by surgeons who had more experience with this procedure.

I realized then that experience is very important in this kind of surgery, and since throat cancer frequency is diminishing in this country, there are fewer patients with this type of cancer and surgeons consequently have less experience removing it. With so few patients, it is no surprise that expertise in its removal and care is concentrated in just a few places. Obviously, my surgeons had very little experience using laser to remove my type of cancer. I was wondering why the department head, the one that used the laser, stated that if he felt that he could not remove my cancer with laser, he would have told me so. I sympathized with his honest self-confidence, because even though I am not a surgeon, I had probably manifested similar self-assurance whenever I talked with patients and their family members. However, as I became older and more experienced, I often admitted my shortcomings and deferred decisions to physicians who were more experienced in areas I was not. Since I liked my surgeons very much,

I ignored consideration of their competence in this procedure when I made my decision to let them operate on me.

I asked the doctors to look for my wife, who was still waiting for me in the ward to take me home. She needed to be informed about the unexpected developments. When she came in, they repeated their explanations and entertained her questions as well. I tried to maintain my composure so that my wife would not be too upset. I even assisted the doctors in explaining the situation to her. It was very difficult and upsetting for her to absorb and understand what had happened and how could it have occurred.

The last thing that I had to deal with was to decide what to do next. I had to make a choice. I could accept the offer of my surgeons to refer me to another center or let them retry remove the cancer. Before I made the decision, I had to absorb and digest the new reality and assess the pros and cones of each choice.

I knew that if I decided to seek care in another center, this would take time and further delay the removal of my cancer. Any other surgeon would have to first assess me and fit me into his or her busy schedule. I also felt weak and tired a week past my surgery. I knew that getting the cancer out of my body without further delay was of utmost importance because it reduced the chances of spreading to other organs. I also thought that my surgeons were the best people to go back into my upper airways, because they were familiar with me, knew what had been done before, and had a specific idea of what needed to be done in order to correct the situation. This territory would be completely new for any new surgeon.

I told my surgeons the truth: I had lost much of my trust in them and, in retrospect, I realize I should have gotten help elsewhere. However, I was going to give them a second chance for two purely selfish reasons. They knew me best, and they were going to remove the cancer in forty-eight hours.

Sharing the situation with my oldest daughter and son who were waiting for me in the hospital ward was not easy, but my wife and I did it in a calm and reassuring way. As a parent, I tried to stay calm and in control so that they would not become too upset. What was done was done. It was now time to move on and plan the next step the best I could. Since there was no available operating room at the Army Hospital until the following week, I was to be discharged home and readmitted to the Navy Hospital a few miles away in two days. Even though I had had so many disappointments and letdowns during my week-long hospitalization, I wished at that time that I could have had the next surgery in the same place so that I would not have to go through the red tape of being discharged and readmitted. However, I thought I could use a short break from being a patient, get a good night's sleep, and finally get rid of my intravenous line. Furthermore, I was more familiar with the Naval Hospital where I had practiced before, had previously been a patient, and knew many more medical personnel. I also felt better going to the hospital that belonged to the service to which I used to belong.

It was a bittersweet discharge from the hospital that took place about nine p.m. that evening. I wished everything would just be over and I would already be cured. However, I had to face and deal with a new reality and a seemingly unending saga of trials.

I picked up my medications from the night pharmacy at the hospital and was escorted to the parking lot by one of the nurses. Even though she did not know me, she gave me a big hug before I entered the car. This was a nice final human touch ending a tumultuous and difficult week.

Chapter 11. Another Attempt

I had only a day and a half to spend at home before the next surgery. I mainly used the time to read my mail and take care of some urgent matters and also digest the events that had transpired in the past week. After more fully integrating the impact of what my doctors had failed to do, I was wondering if such errors were common and if the doctors' plan for the future course of action was logical and adequate. I had developed mistrust and built up a lot of anger and resentment towards them because of their failure to remove the cancer, so much so that I even contemplated pursuing legal action. I was in a peculiar situation because I was going to trust my life to the hands of my surgeons, but at the same time contemplating a malpractice case as an expression of my anger and a wish to prevent such errors in the future. I emailed a lawyer and a physician friend with whom I had previously worked as an expert witness on malpractice cases to tell them what had happened.

An email message from that friend influenced my attitude at the right time when I read it early in the morning before the second surgery:

> "…the key is to succeed tomorrow, and the rest can be discussed later. Good luck. I will think of you and hope that it will all work out. Do not burden yourself with negative thoughts!!! Anyone can miss a lesion. It is regrettable, but not negligent. You need to trust these doctors tomorrow! Think positively!"

115

What he told me was to discard any negative, angry feelings and concentrate my energy toward positive thinking as I was facing the surgery and my ultimate recovery. He also stressed that this was not true and blunt negligence, but failure to detect the real cancer. I also realized that the main consequence of the doctors' mistake was that I needed one extra surgery and still carried the cancer for an additional nine days. These were probably minuscule issues and did not justify pursuing legal action. After thinking about these issues and weighing the options, I chose not to pursue legal action, mostly because I still felt a lot of affection, camaraderie and friendship toward some of these doctors. What I was not aware of at that time was that the best chance to completely remove the tumor using laser was on the first attempt and that every subsequent attempt was going to be more difficult because of the post-surgical changes and swelling that made the use of endoscopy more difficult. This cruel reality became evident later on.

I used the short time between the hospitalizations to update and consult some of the specialists across the country and overseas. I was not sure whether to trust myself at the hands of my surgeons again and needed some perspective from other experts. Many of them responded to me immediately, and one even did it from an overseas trip.

The European laser specialist wrote:

"Missing the tumor during surgery is really a very unhappy event! It may have occurred because your surgeons did not undertake the diagnostic endoscopy, which has been performed in another hospital before. However, I would still recommend removing the tumor by transoral laser surgery. The fact that the lesion has been missed suggests that it is obviously not in an advanced stage and probably well circumscribed. I wish you the very best for the planned revision."

The sender of another email actually called me later from India where he was attending a conference and suggested that I go ahead

116

with the attempt to remove the cancer again by laser, but his initial response to my dilemma was:

"I arrived late last night in Mumbai for a laryngeal conference. It's very late now here in India....

I have read your email now. This is a tough situation. Biopsies of tumors in the radiated field are extremely difficult at times to manage. Was there initially tumor present? It could have been very small and removed in its entirety with the biopsy. It could have been missed. It's hard to say.

Let's assume there's residual disease. If the surgeon can see the residual disease, then re-resection seems appropriate, but it is almost impossible for me to read between all these lines."

I checked into the Navy Hospital early in the morning on the day of surgery, hoping that this time things would work out. I felt more comfortable being admitted to that hospital where I had been a staff member and because I had been admitted there before and always had satisfactory experiences. When I was considering joining the military, I decided to join the Navy rather than the Army, partially because I felt a greater cordiality and comradeship there. The same attitude was also reflected in the Navy Hospital in Bethesda, Maryland. In contrast to my experience at the Army Hospital, the pre-surgical admission process was personal and efficient, and I found myself in separate cubicle where I had my vital signs taken. After being taken to the operating room area, an intravenous infusion was started, and I met the anesthetist and his nurse. The surgeons greeted me before they walked into the operating room, and shortly afterward I was taken there myself.

I woke up in the SICU and learned that the procedure took only four hours. The surgeons informed me that this time, they were successful in removing the cancer using the laser. They were more certain of that because this time they had confirmed that the resected lesion was indeed cancerous by examining a frozen section of the removed tissues right there in the operating room. Furthermore, they assured me that no cancer cells were found in the margins around the tumors. For this reason, no more surgery would be needed, and I was most likely finally free of cancer. However, they reminded me that pathological results of frozen sections were only ninety percent accurate compared to the final ones. The definite readings would become available only in about five days.

This was finally great news! For the first time, I felt elated and optimistic, as did my family. Because I was anaesthetized only for a shorter period of time as compared to my previous surgery, I felt better sooner; and although I had excellent individual nursing at the SICU, I did not require much special care. I was able to sit up and even walk within four to six hours after the surgery. When I walked around the SICU, I realized that I was probably the least sickly patient there.

I was taken to the surgical ward the next day, where I was placed in an individual room. I had an intravenous fluid catheter and was fed again through a nasal tube that again became annoying and painful after a couple of days. The nursing care this time was impeccable and very professional. The staff was very caring and responsive, and I felt very grateful and appreciative to be in an environment where I did not have to be on guard all the time. The only issue I had to deal with was a civilian nurse who was efficient but belligerent at times and had an unfriendly attitude. I simply requested another nurse and never had to deal with the first nurse again.

The residents and staff physicians, who were the same as the ones I had at the other hospital, continued to be very diligent and compassionate and did their best to ease my recovery. I was very touched when my surgeon came one evening to watch with us the premier showing of a documentary movie that was made by my son and was shown on public television. I wanted to believe that the special care and attention I was getting from my surgeon was more than the result of his guilt feelings or fear of legal action. In retrospect, I think that he would have been just as attentive and caring even if he would not have missed the cancer on the first surgery.

I was wondering why was there such an immense difference in the quality of care I had received between the two military hospitals. The only explanation I came up with was that almost all of the nursing staff at the Navy Hospital were relatively young active duty personnel and had uniform training, which they performed to the best of their abilities in a no-nonsense military routine. In contrast, more than half of the staff nurses at the Army Hospital were civilians and generally older. It is very likely that the civilian nurses had been trained at different schools, and being that many were civil service personnel, they did not feel bound by the military codes and strict rules. These rules stress respect and obedience and strict adherence to protocol, including performing medical procedures.

As I recovered slowly, after about five days I was able to resume oral intake and with the encouragement of my son took several daily walks in the hospital corridors. When the day came for my oldest daughter to fly back to California, I encouraged her to do so. Although she wanted to stay longer, I felt that there was no more reason for her to delay her return. I was recovering quickly and, at this hospital, there was no real need for her to watch over me to make sure there were no mistakes.

As the fifth day after my surgery approached, I was expecting to learn about the final pathology report. I was hoping to hear good news that confirmed the initial findings. The report was indeed ready on that day, and one of surgeons delivered it to me. The final reading confirmed that the margins of the tumor were indeed clear of cancer, but the tumor itself was positive all the way to these margins at the lower part of the tumor. This was disconcerting to the surgeons because they were not sure they had removed all of the cancer. To find out if any cancer was left behind, they decided to perform another surgery two days later so that they could remove more tissues at the upper and lower edges of the area where the tumor was previously present. This would be my third weekly surgery, and I was beginning to feel like I was on some bizarre, outlandish weekly surgery regimen.

I felt great disappointment at this news. I had been so reassured by what seemed to be a successful removal of the cancer, only to learn that my saga had no end in sight. I had, however, no choice but to accept this reality. I also felt great gratitude for my doctors who were so diligent and responsible this time and were doing their best to assure that I was finally completely cancer-free. I was hoping that this surgery would be the last and that it would finally end this continuous chase that requires more surgeries.

I was taken to the operating room for my next surgery directly from my hospital bed. This time, the procedure took only two hours, and after a short stay in the recovery room, I was returned to my hospital bed. There were no frozen sections taken this time because the removed tissues were sent in their entirety for thorough pathological studies.

After an additional four days, the final news came back. The tissues at the bottom of the cancer were positive. This meant that the cancer was still in my throat and was acting in an unpredictable way. Even though the margins at that area were negative, the tumor skipped that area and emerged at a different site. This was very unsettling news and meant that further surgery was needed. My surgeons felt that the laser option had been exhausted because the remaining cancer would be very hard to reach using laser. "Therefore," they explained, "the next step will be to perform a more aggressive surgery, the one we had planned to do before – a bigger resection of the entire region, using a flap of tissue from your leg to cover the defect." This surgery was to take place later in the same week, which would ironically be my fourth weekly surgery.

I was discharged again from the hospital and was told to return three days later for the definite surgery. I tried again to digest and accept my situation but found it difficult to accept the failure of the laser surgery to remove the cancer. I was wondering if perhaps I should seek the care of one of the three national specialists in laser surgery. Perhaps one of them could still reach the tumor area where my own surgeons could not.

I contacted all of these experts and was able to talk to two of them. Both were willing to see me in their clinics; one was only able

120

to do that in about three weeks, and the other in a week. Neither was willing to promise that they would be able to assist me until they had examined me.

I also emailed the German world expert in laser surgery who had responded to my queries before. He responded with this honest and clear message agreeing with my surgeons' plan:

"I'm sorry to hear that the laser revision surgery you received was obviously unsuccessful. On principle, the apex of the pyriform sinus is also accessible to transoral laser microsurgery; however, when I recap the treatment approaches during the last weeks, I think that your surgeons may be not experienced enough in the use of the laser. So, I would also recommend now to resect the remaining tumor from outside, because surgery is the only chance you have to get cured. I further think that it wouldn't be a good idea in this situation to change to another doctor who would try laser surgery again. Your surgeons are the only ones who know exactly where tumor tissue is probably still left behind in the pharynx and where a further resection is necessary.

I wish you the best for the next and hopefully last surgical step!"

I felt again most grateful to this expert, whom I knew only by reputation, for repeatedly giving me clear and succinct advice.

I had a pre-surgical meeting with my surgeons where they outlined their planned surgical approach. They recapped their plan and honestly detailed the pitfalls of the procedure and its complications. They also explained that following the surgery, I would have to breathe through a temporary tracheotomy for a few months, may have permanent problems in swallowing, and would have a lifelong high-risk of aspiration of food.

After listening to these explanations, I was able to have a greater appreciation of the consequences of this surgery. Even though I received advice to the contrary, I was still wondering if this extensive surgery was really necessary and if the laser option was completely lost. While I was initially hesitant and unsure about the merits of laser surgery, once I was faced with the more extensive surgery and its permanent results, I refused to abandon the initial option entirely. I wondered if laser surgery might still be a viable tool in the hands of a more experienced surgeon.

Seeking a fresher look at my situation, I asked my surgeons if I could consult one of the experts in laser surgery to make sure I had completed exhausted this option. They were very responsive to my request, put off the planned surgery, and promised to assist me in getting another opinion. They contacted Dr. Roger in Philadelphia an expert in robotic head and neck surgery including the use of laser. I had communicated with Dr. Roger earlier when I was looking for advice. His secretary called me within a few hours to schedule an appointment to see him in his clinic on the following day. I gathered all my medical and pathological records, including a summary that I was provided with, and set out to see the expert early in the morning on the day I was supposed to have my fourth surgery.

Driving to Philadelphia was a more convenient option than flying to the other centers where laser surgery is performed. Although I knew several physicians at the hospital in Philadelphia, including the Chairman of the Department of Otolaryngology, I had no time to contact them before the trip. There was actually no need to contact any of them, because I was going to see Dr. Roger right away. However, knowing that I had acquaintances at that medical center was reassuring. I felt so fortunate to be able to see the specialist without any delay and was most grateful to my surgeons and the secretary at the expert's office for facilitating the visit. I knew that waiting a longer time before getting an appointment would have been very difficult for me. The urgency to get cured was the driving force that kept me going forward and helped me overcome feelings of depression, anger, and exhaustion.

My wife and I left for Philadelphia early the next morning. It was strange to drive through the very familiar route that we had often taken on route to Philadelphia or New York to visit family members.

Driving to Philadelphia for medical reasons was emotionally difficult for my wife, who grew up in that city and had to make such trips when her late parents were terminally ill. We arrived at University Hospital and found our way to the clinic through the maze of rooms and buildings. After a short wait, we were directed through a long corridor lined with a row of small patient rooms into one of them. After about half an hour, a nurse came in to take a detailed medical history and fill out several forms. She did it in a mechanical, non-personal, non-interested manner. Although I had written down the main medical events of the past two years for her, she had great difficulty in understanding the issues and kept making mistakes in the paperwork. I had to explain the history several times before she finally got it correct.

After an additional twenty minutes, a secretary came in to fill out insurance papers asking questions similar to the ones the other nurse had just asked. It was very frustrating to repeat all of these answers, and I was wondering why the information was not taken only once.

After she left, we had to wait twenty minutes more before another medical staff member walked in. She was to spray my nostrils with local anesthetic in preparation for an endoscopic examination. It took a few seconds for me to realize that she was inexperienced in performing the simple procedure, and I had to explain to her how to do it correctly. I was wondering if the topical anesthetic would wear off before Dr. Roger would actually come to examine me. Following this, we were left alone again wondering why we had to wait so much time to see the doctor. I looked outside my cubicle and realized that all the other half dozen rooms in the long corridor were full of patients like me who were also waiting for Dr. Roger to show up. This seemed to be an impersonal mass treatment approach that was obviously created to make it easy for Dr. Roger to see as many patients as possible in the shortest time frame. All the necessary information was taken and preparations were made beforehand to make it easier and quicker for him. There was an aura of great expectation for the "expert" to finally arrive. It felt so impersonal and mechanical.

Finally, he appeared and, after progressing through the long corridor seeing several patients, walked into my room. He was escorted
by an entourage of several junior doctors and a foreign physician who
had come to study under him. Dr. Roger seemed aloof and aware of
his importance, and this made me feel even weaker in my vulnerable physical state. In contrast, the other surgeons I had previously
encountered seemed more personable and humble in nature. I wanted
to share with Dr. Roger my thoughts and criticism of that morning
experiences. However, I was forced to keep silent and subject myself
to this degrading attitude without any complaint because I needed
his help and depended on his willingness to take my case.

He briefly asked me for my medical history, essentially repeating
the same questions the nurse and secretary had taken before. This
suggested to me that he had not even read the history they had taken.
He then proceeded to examine my upper airways and performed an
endoscopic examination. When he concluded, he told us that he could
not visualize the affected area and, in order to do that, he would need
to use direct laryngoscopy performed under general anesthesia. The
advantage of that procedure is that it would enable him to introduce a
larger instrument into my larynx through which he could get a better
view. Only after that would he be able to decide if he could remove
the rest of the cancer.

The secretary scheduled that procedure for the following week,
and I was sent on to have several pre-surgical blood tests. Although
I understood the need to go through another operating room procedure, I was disappointed because I still did not have a clear answer or
plan for removing the tumor.

Before returning to Washington, I decided to visit my friend, the
Chairman of the Department of Otolaryngology. I learned that he had
recently become the dean of the local medical school, and his office
was located now in the medical school building. I wanted to let him
know about my medical problem and hoped that he could assist me
in case I needed any help. I took the elevator to the top floor of the
tower office building adjacent to the hospital and, although I had
not announced my visit, I was fortunate to be able to see him right

away. He had a magnificent view of Philadelphia from his office. He greeted me very warmly, but I could sense that he was troubled and in ill spirits. I understood why very quickly when he proceeded to share with me his own medical problems and the surgery he would soon undergo. I spent most of my time in his office comforting him and wishing him well in preparation for his upcoming surgery. This made me realize that I was not alone with serious medical problems and that being in the medical profession does not protect us.

We returned to Philadelphia five days later on a cold and snowy day. After checking into the hospital, I went through the pre-surgical rituals that I had unfortunately become very familiar with. I changed into hospital clothes and was escorted to the pre-surgical waiting area. The medical staff was efficient and compassionate, which made the process smoother. Shortly afterwards, I was taken to the operating room and put to sleep. I was expecting to be asleep for at least an hour but woke up in a recovery room only thirty minutes later.

I learned why my anesthesia time was so short when Dr. Roger came to see me some time later. He was very brief when he delivered the news. He was unable to visualize the affected area because there was so much post-surgical swelling that his instruments could not even be inserted into my lower airways. "This swelling," he continued, "will prevent me from performing any laser surgery using robotic technique." I realized for the first time that the laser procedures that I endured in the past three weeks had truly left their mark and caused changes that prevent any further use of laser, at least for some time. I also understood that the first time is the best time for laser to be utilized, and any repeat use was going to be more difficult.

Dr. Roger's opinion was that my best option now was to be seen by one of the best head and neck cancer surgeons in the nation, Dr. Marker, who practiced in New York City. Dr. Marker would be able to suggest the best surgical approach. He promised to contact Dr. Marker himself and ask him to see me. Surprisingly, my experience that day with Dr. Roger was more positive, as he acted very responsibly and fulfilled his promise to make sure that I reached the next level of care.

Nevertheless, hearing this news was very disappointing to me. This entirely closed the option of resorting to laser. All my hopes of finally getting someone to take care of the cancer vanished, and I had wasted an additional eight days without any resolution. It was a sad trip back home. On our way back, I received a call from Dr. Roger's secretary to inform me that he had already talked with Dr. Marker, who agreed to see me, and that she would forward all the medical records to him. I called the office of Dr. Marker and was fortunate to get an appointment the next day. Later on, I realized that this detour on the way to getting the final cure was worth it, because even though Dr. Roger was unable to help me, he was instrumental in referring me to the best expert in the field.

Chapter 12. The Definite Surgery

My wife and I arrived at Dr. Marker's New York clinic on a Wednesday afternoon. My youngest daughter also joined us after she finished her work. The clinic is located a few blocks away from the hospital where Dr. Marker operates and is staffed by very efficient and cordial personnel who made the visit as pleasant and personal as possible. The waiting area was crowded, but after a short time, we were taken to a quieter special waiting area in the back.

In the waiting area, I saw several patients who had recent extensive head and neck surgery, as was evident by their appearance and scars. Some patients like me were there for the first time, and others came from out of town, including Europe and Israel. They and their family members looked anxious, just as we probably did. We all had come to seek the help of the expert with a worldwide reputation.

We were directed to a small examination room where we waited for almost an hour before Dr. Marker finally came in. He was very friendly, personable, and knowledgeable and exuded an aura of confidence and genuine care. After listening to my medical history, he proceeded to examine me thoroughly again using endoscopy, reviewed the documents and the radiographic tests that I had brought with me, and proceeded to explain his plan of action. He felt that since the cancer had recurred after receiving radiation, removal of the cancer using laser was not a good option in my case. He believed that since my cancer was behaving in a non-conventional manner, skipping areas that had been scarred after being eradiated, the best option for me now was to undergo the most aggressive kind of surgery. This entailed removing my retropharynx and the entire larynx, including the vocal cords. To reconstruct that area and rebuild an upper digestive tract, he would replace the removed parts by transplanting a flap of skin with its underlying tissues from my hand or thigh. I would no longer be able to breathe through my nose or mouth because he would redirect the trachea so that it would open in my neck, creating a tracheotomy.

He also brought up the issue of alternative ways by which I could still be able to speak – information I had previously heard from my surgeons in Washington. He told me that immediately after the surgery, I would not be able to speak and would have to communicate by writing. After my upper airways were healed, I could try to speak through a voice prosthesis. He told me that an SLP who works with him would meet with me after he finished and educate me and provide more detailed information about my speech rehabilitation.

His voice and demeanor were very confident and assertive, which left no doubt in me that he was right. I realized that he did not believe in the use of laser surgery as an alternative to extensive surgery, but at that juncture, after laser had failed to work for me, I was willing to accept his plan. Yet this was devastating news. I was hoping that what Dr. Marker would suggest would be a less radical kind of surgery in order to preserve my vocal cords.

Accepting that I would have my vocal cords removed was easier for me than I had previously thought it would be. I have seen individuals who had laryngectomy before, and I always felt very sorry for them and thought, *If that was me, I would never agree to lose my vocal cords. I'd die first.* However, when I actually had to face this reality, I agreed without any hesitation. After what I had endured in the past two months, I was ready to accept this treatment. Increasing my chance to live was worth this price. I realized that I had no other recourse, and even if this option failed, at least I would know that I tried to do the best to remove the cancer.

Dr. Marker also stressed that he could not predict how much of the cancer was still present in my throat and that it was quite possible that only very little of it was left after my previous surgeries. However, I knew that even a few cells of this tumor could still kill me if left behind and that my best chance of living was to undergo the extensive surgery he recommended. There was no doubt in my mind that this had to be done. Agreeing to his plan, I urged him to schedule me for surgery as soon as possible. I strongly felt the urgency to get the cancer out without further delay.

Dr. Marker proceeded to explain the surgery and the time I would spend in the hospital afterwards. After the surgery, I would spend about two days in the SICU and then be moved to the Otolaryngology Ward, first to the Step-Down Unit (a specialized unit where more intensive care is given) and then to the regular ward. I would be fed through a tube for two weeks until the transplanted tissues were integrated, and then I would carefully start eating by mouth.

We had asked him numerous questions to try to clarify some of the issues that were unclear, but there were many more that we did not think of until later. We called his office a few days later with some other questions, which one of his associates answered. After Dr. Marker explained the special care that needed to be taken to prevent the transplanted tissues from failing and the delicacy of the blood supply to it, I realized that my migraine headache medication (which works by constricting the blood vessels) might interfere with the blood supply to transplanted tissues. He agreed with my concerns and referred me to a pain specialist to look for alternative medications. Unfortunately, that would require an additional trip to New York because there were no available appointments until the following week.

We met with the SLP for more than an hour, and she explained the options I would have to speak again. She was very friendly, patient, and extremely knowledgeable and worked very closely with Dr. Marker. Listening to her made me feel that I was going to be taken care of by an excellent and experienced team that would guide me through the difficult future.

There was so much information that I had to absorb that day, and I had trouble digesting all of it. Even though I heard and understood them, the facts were still so abstract, and I did not truly understand their full impact and consequences. When I finally had to face these life-changing realities, I realized that there was so much more information I did not hear about – even facts I heard felt so different when I actually experienced them. I realized later that no preparation can make one truly ready for these events.

The news was very hard to digest. My daughter started crying, and I had to comfort and console her and explain why this was the best and only option left for me. I had to be strong for her and my family, even though the news was devastating. I knew that by staying strong and doing the best to get cured – even though what was waiting for me was a difficult road – I was setting an example for my children that a person should not give up and needs to keep fighting, even in the face of adversity. *They are young,* I thought, *but one day they may have to face similar issues.* This motivation kept me strong and helped me overcome the lows and hardships I would experience in the coming months.

After finishing the necessary paperwork and filling out several forms, we met with the scheduling nurse who set a date for the surgery five weeks later. It was disappointing to have to wait so long. It was clear that Dr. Marker was extremely busy, and his schedule was full. He was so popular and was sought by so many patients that such a wait was to be expected. However, the nurse promised to do her best to try to advance my case if possible. This would be possible, she explained, if a cancellation occurred or if another patient would be willing to give up their turn for me. I badly wanted this to happen, as waiting so much time seemed very difficult.

We left the clinic more than six and a half hours later. Time went by quickly and intensely. I was surprised that the staff was not urging us to leave until they took care of everything and all our questions were answered and needs were met. I felt I was in good hands and we were very grateful to receive so much care and consideration in these challenging times. It was new for me to be taken care of in a civilian hospital after getting all of my previous medical care in military hospitals. I was a little apprehensive about being taken care of by physicians I had not previously known or worked with. On the other hand,

I was happy that my three children who lived in New York would not have to travel to Washington to be with me during the surgery. Even though I was exhausted, I finally had true hope that the definitive surgery would finally take place, and I would become cancer-free. I was fighting for my chance to live.

I returned to Washington expecting a long wait before I was to come back to New York for my surgery. While in Washington, I was still recovering from my recent operations and had to deal with throat discomfort and pain. A few days after my return, I started to experience increased pain in the middle of my chest and slight fever. My local surgeons were concerned that I had developed an infection of the mediastinal space, which is very serious and one of the complications of the type of surgeries I had. They admitted me to the hospital and gave me antibiotics to combat the potential infection but, fortunately, further tests excluded this complication, and I was happy to go back home after only one day.

I had mixed feelings about having to wait so long for the next surgery. On the one hand, I appreciated the respite from hospitalizations and the return to "normal" life, but I wanted to get cured as soon as possible and knew that the cancer could still spread during this time.

The following week, I returned to New York to be examined by a pain specialist at the same building where I saw Dr. Marker. He gave me a most thorough physical and neurological examination and suggested several anti-migraine medications for me to try before the surgery. After the visit, my son and I walked around the neighborhood a little, and I thought that it might be a good idea for me to visit the hospital prior to the surgery. It occurred to me that getting familiar with the place might be useful to reduce my anxiety.

The hospital was located in a relatively underdeveloped neighborhood in Manhattan, and I was surprised to find that the building was old and shabby. There was no main hall at the entrance, and the layout of the wards was very confusing and difficult to navigate. I specifically looked for the admitting and family waiting areas, the operating rooms, the SICU, and the hospital floor where I would be admitted. I wanted to see all these places prior to the surgery so I could navigate with ease afterwards. I found out where I should go on the day of my surgery, where my family would wait, and how the otolaryngology floor looked. I did not want to be surprised when I woke up from the anesthesia. After concluding the tour, I felt that I was more prepared for the upcoming hospitalization.

Seeing the poor condition of the hospital was disappointing for me because I was used to working in a much more modern facility and had visited other medical centers in New York City which were more modern and looked more attractive. However, I reminded myself that I should not judge the place by its looks and what I was coming here for was to get an excellent surgical care. Although it is nice to be hospitalized in pleasant surroundings, what is actually more important is the quality of care.

My doctors in Washington suggested that I use my time to get prepared for the aftermath of the laryngectomy by meeting their hospital SLP and also two individuals who had had such surgery. The SLP was a young and enthusiastic individual who was very eager to help and exhibited great self-confidence. Although I did not realize at that time how important a competent and helpful SLP is for recovery and adjustment to life after laryngectomy, meeting her made me feel more confident about the support system I would have.

I met patients who had had laryngectomy at the Otolaryngology Clinic at the hospital. Meeting these patients was very informative and useful but, in retrospect, it was difficult for me at that time to fully accept the notion that I would soon become one of them. The idea that I was about to lose my vocal cords was too abstract to comprehend. Even though I knew this intellectually, it seemed surreal at that time.

The first laryngectomee had the procedure about eight years earlier and seemed very adapted to his situation. He spoke using a voice prosthesis and came to the clinic to change it. My wife and I watched the SLP take the old device out and insert the new one. The procedure seemed simple and only took a few minutes, but watching the patient's face seemed to indicate that he experienced some discomfort.

When I first watched his tracheotomy stoma, through which I could visualize the inside of the trachea, I was taken aback. It looked raw and very exposed to the outside world.

The quality of the laryngectomy patient's voice was relatively good, which was reassuring to me, and he seemed to be well-adapted to this speech form. He told us about his past difficulties and the personal and psychological hardships he endured and how depressed he had become after his surgery. What was reassuring to hear was that he eventually overcame these issues and was more content at present. He graciously offered to personally assist me by email or phone if I would want to correspond. He kept his promise and wrote to me several times after my surgery and offered his advice and encouragement.

A few days later, we met the second patient who is the president of the local Laryngectomee Club. He came especially to meet me, as it was his custom to pay a visit to each of the future laryngectomee in the Greater Washington region. I learned later that the SLPs in the region knew about his important services and his dedication to helping potential patients learn to cope with the consequences of losing their vocal cords. He spoke using an electro-larynx, which produced a very strong background sound that made listening and understanding difficult. Since we had never heard anyone speak in that fashion, it was initially very difficult for me to get used to the quality of his voice. However, to my surprise, I became used to his mode of speaking within a short period of time and after a while did not even notice its unique nature.

He was very gracious and informative and told us his own personal story and how he had adjusted to living and working with an artificial voice. It was an amazing story that was very inspirational and very useful later on. He brought with him brochures and even supplies that I might need after my surgery and invited me to join the local club and come to their meetings even before my surgery. I initially thought that I would go to the meeting prior to my surgery but decided not to do so at that time. I thought that seeing individuals who had lost their vocal cords would be too upsetting to me, and I also did not want the attendees to see me with normal voice while they themselves were without. However, this club (and especially its president) played a major role in my recuperation later on. His enthusiastic support and availability at all times were unsurpassed.

The long wait for the surgery fortunately ended sooner than I anticipated. About three weeks after my first visit to Dr. Marker, on a Thursday afternoon, I received a call from his nurse coordinator that there was an available opening for surgery the next day or on the upcoming Tuesday. One of the patients who had a non-urgent procedure the following week was willing to swap with me. I was very grateful for the opportunity to finally undergo the surgery but elected to wait until the following week to have it done. Undergoing surgery the following day was too immediate, and I did not want to recover from a serious surgery over the weekend when the hospital is manned only by on-call physicians. My medical experience had taught me that it is more difficult to access the best medical care during weekends or holidays.

A couple of days before the operation, I was contacted by one of Dr. Marker's assistants, whose job was to help the patients and their families. She offered practical advice regarding the day of surgery and told me where my family could wait during the operation. She was warm and compassionate and proved to be a great asset for me and my family throughout the hospitalization. Getting that call was most reassuring and provided a personal touch to the upcoming hospitalization.

We arrived in New York a day prior to the surgery. This was a very somber and serious period when I was apprehensive, nervous, and quietly worried about the complicated surgery and its aftermath. I was told in the afternoon that I was scheduled to be the second surgical case the following day and should arrive in the hospital at eleven a.m. I was not happy to be the second case because I was afraid that my surgeon might be tired by the time he operated on me and also because it required me to fast for more hours. However, the nurse coordinator explained that Dr. Marker leaves the more complicated cases to the end of the day because then he is not constraint by any time limitations. Furthermore, she assured me that Dr. Marker is never tired and can work until late without any difficulties.

In the afternoon, I went with my son and granddaughter to Central Park, where she had great fun climbing rocks and using the swings – a last chance for some fun before the big day.

We stayed with my daughter the night before the surgery. Before leaving her apartment on the morning of the surgery, I made sure I did not carry my wallet or watch with me and brought only essential documents such as my Medicare and military retiree identification cards. My daughter drove all of us to the hospital and, as we approached, I realized that what was waiting for me was getting closer and closer. Fortunately, once we arrived in the hospital, all my initial trepidations were overcome by a determination to get the task done. Getting started with the final process of admission was a good distraction from the worries.

Since I had previously visited the hospital, I knew how to quickly find the admission area. It was a very crowded and uncomfortable room, and after a short wait, I was asked to go to an adjacent room where I had to fill out some paperwork. I brought with me the legal documents where I named my wife and son as those who could make medical decisions in case I was incapacitated. The bureaucratic process was very impersonal, and after its conclusion, I was directed to an area where I had to change into hospital clothes. My vital signs were taken, and after a short stay, a nurse came to take me to the operating room preparation area. I asked her for permission to say goodbye to my family. I quickly walked to the waiting area where I hugged and kissed them and reminded them to wait in the specially designated area for head and neck surgery family members where the surgeons would inform them about the progress of the operation. I did not even think at that moment that this was the last time I would speak with them in my normal voice.

I was taken to the operating room floor where I was directed to a surgical bed. The waiting time was unnerving. After a while, one of the surgeons whom I had not previously met walked by and talked with me for a few minutes. He was very friendly and kind, which eased my anxiety a little. Some time later, an anesthetist briefly examined me and started an intravenous infusion. He explained that he would later introduce an arterial line into my groin area to monitor my blood pressure and perform other functions as needed. My surgeon also came in for a short time and quickly returned to the operating room.

A short time later, I was wheeled to the operating room through a long corridor. The operating room was quite empty compared to the one in the Army hospital, and there was only a single nurse there when I arrived. I was asked to lie down on the operating table, and the nurse started to prepare me for surgery. After a short while, the anesthetist and a colleague of my surgeon walked in. I had not met that surgeon before, but he was very kind and supportive. When he asked me if I was concerned about anything, I replied that I was worried about the outcome of the surgery and hoped to wake up at the end of it. He smiled and patted me on the shoulder, assuring me that I would wake up and that they would do their best to ensure that the surgery would be a success. With these parting words, the anesthetics began to administer the anesthetic medication into my vein, and I slipped into deep sleep.

Chapter 13. The Surgical Intensive Care Unit Experience

I woke up more than fifteen hours after the surgery. Similar to what I had experienced after the previous long surgery, my recollection of the first few hours after waking up was vague, gradually improving in the ensuing hours. In contrast to my previous surgeries when I stayed in SICU for one to two days, this time I stayed for four. I later learned that the surgery took only about five hours. This was much shorter than the estimated time this surgery would have taken if it would have been done in any of the military hospitals. Even though it was a complex surgery that involved removing my larynx and replacing it with a graft taken from my wrist, thus demanding detailed micro-surgery, the shorter time was an indication of how much more experience the New York team had in performing this complex surgery as compared to the other team. This was good news, because a shorter surgery time has many advantages, as longer anesthesia carries more complications and a higher the risk of infections.

My wife told me that she and my children had been sitting in a special waiting area adjacent to the Otolaryngology Ward for the entire duration of the surgery. They had two visits by members of the surgical team; first by a resident about three hours into the surgery, and the second by Dr. Marker himself at its conclusion. The resident informed them that the operation was proceeding as planned and that I was doing fine. Dr. Marker described to them what was done and assured them that everything went without problems and that they could briefly visit me in SICU. They spent a few minutes with me at the SICU and returned the next morning. I was fortunate that my family members were with me every day from about nine a.m. to nine or ten p.m. They were very devoted and caring, and I had to insist that they leave the hospital at night so that they could get some rest.

I found myself in the SICU in a small cubicle that I later learned was at the end of a very large room. The SICU was very crowded, busy, and noisy. As I was gradually feeling better, the noise and commotion in the SICU became annoying, and I found it difficult to rest and sleep. There were irritating noises that were generated by communication and monitoring equipment that went on day and night, never seeming to stop. I was attended by a nurse who also took care of several other patients. The nurse was often called to care for others that were in greater need than me, and consequently, I was left without anyone most of the time. This was different from my experiences at my previous hospitalizations, when I had one-on-one nursing care in the SICU – a very unfortunate difference because, this time, I needed a lot of individual care.

As expected, I had no ability to speak because my entire larynx – including my vocal cords – was removed. My only way to communicate was by writing everything down. Surprisingly, the hospital had no tools that could help me communicate. Fortunately, in preparation for my hospitalization, my family brought a small whiteboard and erasable markers. I used it to write down whatever I wanted to say and showed it to others to read, hoping they would understand. It was hard to use this method because my left hand was bandaged, and the intravenous line was inserted into my right arm. I frequently misplaced the marker and eraser and also had great difficulty erasing what I had previously written. The markers dried up often, and I sometimes found myself without any form of communication. I was hoping to be attended by patient and understanding staff members, and even though most nurses were patient and waited for me to write down my remarks, some seemed too busy to accommodate that.

My wife told me that the SICU was very crowded and had patients from many countries who spoke different languages. She also told me that most of the other patients in the SICU looked much sicker than I, many were non-communicative, and several were connected to life support equipment. One night, I overheard the events that transpired at the bedside of the patient next to me who was in very critical condition. The patient was from a different country, and the family apparently debated in Spanish (which I did not understand) as to whether or not to agree with the doctor's recommendation to disconnect him from life support. A priest was also involved in counseling them. After initial disagreement between the family members, they finally agreed to stop the supportive therapy, and the patient subsequently died.

It was strange to observe what was happening to a very sick patient, not as a physician but as a patient who was also very frail and at risk of things going wrong. In retrospect, I should have felt strong emotions of fear and apprehension about the possibility of something similar happening to me, but I was apparently too drugged and weak and felt only a sense of apathy and helplessness. I numbly considered the thought of death in an SICU as an acceptable reality.

I was very tired and received pain medication on the first days after surgery, which contributed to my lightheadedness. The intensity of my feelings and emotions was inhibited to a large extent in the earlier days. The main emotions I felt were frustration about my new realities, which included my inability to speak, move my body parts, communicate with others, sense a portion of my neck and face, eat by mouth, or breathe through my nose. As I slowly regained my strength, my awareness of these became more acute.

I became very dependent on others for my needs. I also expected my family members to understand my needs and even predict them at times without even telling them what I wanted or needed. I became frustrated and angry at times when they failed to understand me. Over time, my wife and my youngest daughter began to understand lip reading, which made it easier for me to communicate. However, in the beginning, it was very difficult for them to deal with me.

Getting my body sponged and cleaned by the nurses was very strange for me. Even though I was embarrassed to be washed by another person, I appreciated the fresh feeling that I felt afterwards. I was taught how to wash patients in their beds when I was in medical school in an elective course I took in nursing, and I had washed many patients myself when I worked as a nurse during my years as a medical student. This made it easier for me to help and cooperate with the nurses; however, I never thought I would be the one getting a sponge bath.

The tracheostomy tube that was connected to oxygen and all the bandages on my neck, hand, and thigh restricted my movement in bed. I was lying down on my back and had a very limited ability to move my head from side to side. Even though I could move my hands, I was restricted by the intravenous line. Since I had a urinary catheter and arterial line inserted in my groin, I could not move other parts of my body. As was the case after the previous surgeries, both my legs were wrapped with special inflatable cuffs that were intermittently filled with air every fifteen seconds. This was to prevent the formation of venous clots that can prove deadly. However, the constant pumping of air kept me from falling asleep for hours. I eventually learned to free my legs from these cuffs but made sure to move my muscles repeatedly as a substitute. This way, I could finally fall asleep.

I experienced the same difficulties in falling asleep that I had after each of the previous surgeries. Every time I was about to fall asleep, I started to sense a tingling sensation in my throat that induced coughing. This occurred when saliva started to accumulate in my mouth because I was unable to swallow it while sleeping. Attempting to swallow woke me up. This cycle of coughing and attempting to fall asleep kept happening again and again. Since I no longer breathed through my mouth, this did not interfere with my air intake as it had before. To avoid the need to swallow the saliva, I constantly used a suction catheter to clear my secretions. I tried to leave the catheter in my mouth while attempting to fall asleep, but this did not work very well because it kept falling out. I experimented with several methods to solve this problem, but all my improvisations failed. I finally was able to get some sleep sitting up in my bed and leaning slightly forward so that the saliva would drip out of my mouth into a towel without waking me up. Overall, I spent many hours sleeping, but gradually felt stronger and able to stay awake longer.

I experienced many new and unusual sensations in my mouth, the result of the extensive surgery that removed parts of my neck and replaced them with a flap made of other tissues. These sensations included pain and tingling and a new fullness that I had not experienced before. I even had a strange irritating sensation in the deep back of my throat. This was very annoying and made me cough constantly. I envisioned that this might be the result of some sutures that connected the transplanted flap with what was left of my upper airways. When I wrote about these strange sensations to one of the senior surgeons, he did not explain their origin and bluntly told me, "Get used to strange and new sensations... you're going to have many."

This doctor responded to my concerns in a very annoyed "Do not bother me with irrelevant questions... just accept it quietly" tone of voice. What he failed to understand was that, especially as a physician, this nonchalant attitude was not enough for me. His lack of interest in what I sensed showed complete lack of understanding of what was happening to me and left me in the dark regarding what might have been causing the symptoms. For him, I was just one more case who would eventually get better and adjust, and there was no need for him to spend more time explaining the details. But for my part, as a physician, I wanted to know why I was having these sensations – not just that I would have them. To make it even harder, I could not speak up or get his attention again as he quickly moved to the next patient.

I realized in that moment that it was easier for me to accept symptoms and new findings as long as I could understand their origins. What I had wished was that he would explain to me the cause of my symptoms, as he knew what was done to me during the surgery and what the likely consequences of those procedures were. As a physician, it was in my nature and my training to attempt to understand what is behind every situation and finding. It had been my custom to always explain to my patients the science and logic behind any symptom or condition they had. As a patient, I often came up with an explanation myself, but since all of these symptoms were new to me and I had minimal experience in neck surgery, I sometimes envisioned explanations that were incorrect and caused me unnecessary alarm and worry. Unfortunately, most of the surgeons that treated me were not interested in giving me explanations and just brushed my inquiries off. This, of course, only served to increase my frustration and anxiety.

I was also taken care of by a consulting internist who made almost daily bedside visits throughout my hospitalization, mostly to adjust my caloric intake and modify my diet. He was more responsive to my questions and always came up with explanations in areas of his expertise. At times, I even had hard time understanding all of his explanations, partially because I was too worn out to comprehend them. He had also shown more patience in waiting for me to write down my questions, and at times, we carried lengthy dialogs on medical conditions and even on research topics. After my discharge, I emailed him several of my publications on the topics we discussed, and he reciprocated with his.

Fortunately, I was able to find solutions to some of the annoying problems I experienced by using logic and trial and error. One example was dealing with the new symptom I noticed of pain that I felt whenever I swallowed my saliva. I found out that when I leaned to the left while swallowing, the pain significantly decreased. I explained to myself, *This simple method works because it diverts the saliva to an area that is away from the cancer site where there might have been more sutures.* Of course, that was just an unproven theory, but finding an explanation encouraged me to try to help myself whenever I could. Even when I found a physician who would read my questions about the new sensations in my throat, he could not offer me a satisfactory explanation, probably because he did not know what it felt like to have his larynx removed and reconstructed.

Throughout my stay in the SICU, I was lying in a surgical bed completely restricted in movement not only by my pain and neck stiffness, but also by the multiple lines, tubes, and instruments I was connected to. I was hooked up to two infusion lines; one arterial for blood pressure monitoring that was inserted into my right groin, and a venous line for fluids and medications which was placed in my left arm. I was hooked also to several monitoring systems; one for recording my electrocardiogram, which included electrodes on my chest and abdomen; and the other to determine the blood oxygen saturation using a sensor placed on the tip of my finger. I also had a urinary catheter that drained the urine into a collecting bag. I was breathing through a tracheostomy tube inserted into a newly-created opening in my trachea in the middle of my upper chest. The air I was inhaling was mixed with oxygen and humidified by passing through a special bottle with water.

I had several bandaged areas after the surgery: my neck was wrapped snugly, my left arm had a cast and a bandage, and my left thigh was covered with transparent plastic under which was a raw denuded skin. The surgeons had removed the entire larynx and lower pharynx and the lymph glands at the left side of my neck. The lymph gland on the right side had been previously taken out during my first operation. They replaced the removed larynx with tissues from my left arm, folded into a tube-like structure and connected it to my mouth and esophagus. They filled up the defect created in my left arm with skin obtained from my left thigh.

The transplanted tissue (also called "a free flap") was made of the superficial forearm skin and the deeper layers underneath it. The original blood vessels to the flap had to be cut off and reconnected to the blood system in the neck in a very delicate procedure using microscopic surgery. The outcome of the surgery depended on the successful re-implantation of the flap into the neck. The main cause for a flap's failure to integrate in the new place is an interruption in its blood supply that usually occurs in the first two days after the surgery. If failure should occur, the flap has to be immediately accessed and perhaps salvaged. If the flap is not salvageable, it has to be removed and replaced by another. I was told that this is a rare complication, but to detect it early, the free flap would be constantly monitored.

To assure adequate monitoring, a coin-sized tag of skin – part of the hidden interior flap – was left bulging out of the skin in the left side of my neck. Once an hour for the first forty-eight hours, once every two hours for the following forty-eight hours, and less frequently later, the bulging piece of the flap had to be pricked with a needle to see if it bled adequately. If the blood supply was interrupted, the stabbed skin tag would not bleed adequately, which would immediately alert the surgeons to perform an emergency surgery.

I had to endure the repeated checks for the vitality of the flap for the duration of my hospital stay and was relieved each time to hear that it had not failed. Fortunately the needle pricking did not hurt me because the skin tag had no sensation. On several occasions, I had to remind the staff to check it when they were late in doing this. Most of the physicians were familiar with the procedure, but on one occasion, an experienced examiner could not be found, and it took more than forty minutes to find one.

When the bandages around my neck were removed for inspection after forty-eight hours, I realized that in addition to the right side of my neck, I had also lost all sensation to the left side. All perception was missing up to my chin and earlobes and, consequently, I had a scarf-sized area in the front of my neck with no innervations. It was explained to me that when the lymph glands were excised, the sensory nerves that ran through them were also taken out. Immediately after my surgery, I found the lack of sensation very strange and difficult to get used to. Even today, on a cold winter day, I cannot feel the wind blowing on my neck and have to remember to cover it to prevent frostbite. I also have to use an electric razor to shave because when I use a regular blade razor, I often cut myself.

The surgical stitches looked fine but had to be manually debrided and cleaned with hydrogen peroxide and were to be removed in stages. Dr. Marker asked a newly hired nurse to do that. Unfortunately, I learned the hard why she was not a very competent nurse, for she caused me great discomfort in performing the cleaning. She had limited practical experience and trouble holding the surgical instruments, and was moving very slowly. After she repeatedly failed to adequately clean the sutures and made numerous technical mistakes on several other occasions, I finally requested that she no longer care for my wounds. Although I was initially reluctant to express my concern, I eventually learned not to acquiesce when inexperienced or incompetent staff members struggled with simple procedures like cleaning my sutures. I wrote messages to the nurse supervisor or the residents and asked them to have a different nurse perform these chores.

Deciding to assert myself and demand better care came gradually. Initially, I avoided doing so because I felt very dependent and vulnerable and was apprehensive of expressing my dissatisfaction. I was afraid that doing so might upset the staff and cause my care to suffer. I also did not want to cause any professional harm to the nurse if I complain about her shortcomings. However, as I became stronger, I felt that I should not have to put up with situations and performances that made me suffer needlessly. I asked for the change in personnel politely, but also with determination.

The care of my left arm and thigh was labor-intensive and delicate and was done by a resident physician at least twice a day in the first post-surgical week and once a day or more often when needed later. When I first saw my left arm after the cast was removed about two days after the surgery, I noticed that it had a 10 x 6-centimeter deep skin defect at the site where the flap was taken. This had been created because the flap included not only the skin, but also deeper layers. The area from which the flap was taken was covered by a thin skin layer that was harvested from my left thigh, but since that skin missed the deeper layers, it did not fill up the defect. The new transplanted skin that covered the area as well as the skin in front and on one side of it had no sensation. This happened because the new skin was not supplied by any local nerves and also because the nerves that ran through the removed area supplied the other areas around it. The transplanted skin had to be integrated into the arm and was protected from infection by antiseptic bandages that were changed daily.

The missing skin in my left thigh created a raw area that was covered by a transparent bandage that kept being filled up with serous secretions and formed a large bleb of fluid. Because the accumulated fluid tended to break through the cover and leak out, the bandage had to be protected from bursting open at all times. The area was allowed to heal on its own, and the process took almost eight weeks.

My airways had to be repeatedly suctioned by the nurses because I had little strength to cough out the normal secretions it produced. These secretions are always produced by the lungs and are coughed out and swallowed by everyone all the time. However, after laryngectomy, the airways are no longer connected to the mouth, and the only way to clear the tracheal secretions is to cough or suction them out through the opening of the trachea in the neck. Initially, I did not know how to cough through my new orifice. I could not breathe adequately without the suctioning, and sudden blockage of my airways occurred frequently. I was very dependent on these suctions, and since I did not have a nurse by my side at all times (not like in the SICU at the previous hospitals), I often had to call for her by pressing the CALL button and anxiously wait for the nurse to arrive.

Most of the time, the nurse responded within a reasonable period of time, but sometimes there was an extensive delay before the nurse came. On one occasion, I experienced a sudden obstruction of my airway but could not locate the CALL button. It had fallen to the floor because the nurse had not fastened it adequately to my bed when she had made my bed. I tried to get the attention of the staff, but even though I was only a few feet away from the nurses' station, no one seemed to notice my distress. In a desperate attempt to get attention and help, I disconnected the device that monitored my oxygen saturation. I was expecting someone to notice that something was wrong with me because my low reading would generate an alarm in the nurses' station. After no one responded, I disconnected some of the electrocardiogram electrodes. This did not work either. *How can this be ignored in a SICU?* I asked myself. *No heartbeats on the nurses' screens should alert someone!* Fortunately, my wife happened to arrive about ten minutes later and alerted the staff to my condition. This was an awful and scary experience for me. I was helpless getting assistance without a voice and was desperately in need of air while medical personnel simply passed me by and ignored the warning signs that my vitals might be failing.

When my wife went to the nurses' station to complain about what happened, she was rudely rebuffed by the SICU attending physician, who told her not to interfere with his medical rounds. I insisted that the incident be reported to the nurse supervisor, but even when she showed up a few hours later, she did not seemed to be concerned and explained that my nurse was busy caring for other patients. I was too sick to pursue the matter any further. When I brought out this incident to the attention of Dr. Marker, he just shrugged his shoulders and told me that he had little influence on what transpired in the SICU, but he assured me that things would be much better for me when I was moved to the otolaryngology floor where he ran things. He told me that the staff there was more familiar with patients with my kind of operation, so the care there would be much better and more customized to my needs. I could not wait for it to happen.

I received nutrition and oral medication through a thin feeding tube inserted into my esophagus through the tracheostomy opening (stoma). The tube was threaded through a newly created puncture (TEP) that connected the trachea and the esophagus. The tube was held in place by sutures inserted into the skin of my upper chest. Initially, this tube was more convenient than the nasal tube I had after my previous surgeries, but the sutured skin sites started to irritate me and became inflamed after a few days. I was fed every four hours with liquid food that quenched my hunger. It was strange to wait anxiously for this kind of food. It was a relief to eventually be weaned off this mode of feeding and get regular food again.

My blood pressure was very elevated during the first two days after the surgery, and I was putting out a very large volume of urine. I was told that I had received large quantities of fluid during the operation and was getting medications to lower my blood pressure and also get rid of the excessive fluids. After about thirty-six hours, I noted that I was no longer producing so much urine and also felt a sensation of dryness in my mouth. This indicated to me that I had probably gotten rid of the excess fluid in my body. I had made it a habit to ask the nurse what medication I was receiving, so when she was about to intravenously give me a large dose of a urine producing drug, I stopped her from doing so and insisted that she check first with the physician. I did not need help producing more urine at that point. When the physician came he agreed with me that I no longer needed that medication, as my blood chemistry and other tests confirmed that there was no longer a need for it. I felt fortunate to have prevented this over-medication that could have produced untoward side effects. I assumed that such mistakes take place all the time in the busy and impersonal hospital setting.

As I began to feel stronger, I got more involved in checking what medication I was getting. I realized that I was not receiving the correct medication for reduction of my stomach acid production. I had used that drug for several years after others did not work for me. Even though I informed my doctors, anesthetist, and nurses numerous times prior to the surgery what maintenance drugs I was on, they prescribed a different and less effective medication for this. Getting an adequate acid-reducing medication was very important after the surgery because the stomach acidity could reach the operated area in my throat and interfere with the healing of the surgical sutures. But getting the right drug delivered to me proved to be an ordeal.

The resident on call could not prescribe it because the pharmacy refused to dispense it, claiming that it was not covered by Medicare. Finally, after much arm twisting that involved the attending physician, I received the correct medication a day later.

When I inquired if there was an order in my chart that would allow me to receive an anti-migraine medication should I need it, I was told that no such order was written. I was told that even though this was a non-narcotic agent, it could only be prescribed by a pain medication specialist. I had asked the doctors prior to the surgery to have that order on board in case I got a migraine, but they failed to act on it. This was especially frustrating since I had traveled to New York a few weeks before my operation to be examined by a pain management specialist to prepare for such an occurrence and was hoping his recommendations would be followed. I was very concerned that I would suffer from migraines after this surgery, just as I had following my previous ones. When a pain specialist finally arrived a day later, he told me that he could not prescribe a medication for pain that does not exist and those anti-migraine medications are only prescribed by a neurologist. I gave up at this point, as I was too tired and preoccupied with other issues. I just hoped that I would not get a migraine. Fortunately, I had no migraines during the hospitalization.

One of the strange and annoying things that I experienced at the SICU and later on the ward was the accessibility to television. Although every SICU and ward bed had access to an accompanying television set, the use of it was not free and there was a daily charge of ten dollars. A special hospital clerk made daily rounds to ensure that each patient properly apply for and pay for their use of the TV sets by credit card. I had never experienced such a charge in any hospital before and was surprised that the hospital administration was undertaking such desperate measures to look for an extra way to make money, as if the hefty charges of thousands of dollars per day were not enough. It was shameful to watch the money collector pass through the SICU floor soliciting business from very sick patients and their families. Even five-star hotels do not charge their guests for the use of television. Even though I had never applied for television use, I received a bill from the hospital to pay for its use. My wife had to call the Accounting Department to have the charges cancelled.

Being Jewish, I was looking forward to being hospitalized in a hospital with a Jewish name that was founded by Jewish doctors. I thought that I would have the opportunity to be visited by a rabbi, as I had been visited by one during my previous hospitalizations in the military hospitals. Even though I am not very religious, it meant a lot for me to see a rabbi, especially on Friday afternoon before Shabbat. I tried to get a rabbi to visit me, but this proved just as fruitless as my quest for migraine medication, so I finally gave up.

One event that enlightened me during my SICU stay, however, was a story my son told me when he visited me on a Friday afternoon. Before he walked into the hospital to see me, he stopped at a small take-out restaurant near the hospital. The Jewish owner suggested that he try the soup, and when he poured him a bowl, my son realized that he did not carry enough cash to pay for it. The owner told him not to worry about paying for the soup and to pay for it the following week after Shabbat was over. I was so touched by this humane gesture and trust, and I confirmed with my son a few days later that he had paid his debt. I suppose in some way my illness and my dependency on the help of others during my hospital stays had made me more open to noticing and realizing acts of random kindness.

As I gradually regained some strength, I began to integrate what had happened to me and how my life would be different now. I had not previously imagined how I would feel after this major surgical procedure. The pain, weakness, medicated feeling, inability to eat or drink by mouth (I repeatedly dreamed about eating forbidden food), complete dependency, staying connected to an intravenous line, needing humidified oxygenated air, constant suctioning to relieve sudden airway obstruction, having blood drawn almost daily, and being unable to talk were extraordinarily difficult obstacles to adapt to. I understood for the first time why some patients elect to avoid heroic measures to prolong their lives when their prognosis is poor. This was a new realization for me, because I have always believed in prolonging life as long as possible and have tried to practice this principle as a physician. However, I now understood why, at a certain point, this may not be best for some individuals.

I faced the lack of preparation for dealing with some of the issues during my hospitalizations. I had no insight into how or why I was being suctioned. I received different messages and experienced various techniques by different nurses. In contrast to the general similarity in performing procedures and adherence to regulation in the military hospitals, there was significant variability in the private hospital. This was most probably because the nurses at that hospital had been trained by different schools and institutions all over the world. The variability became even more confusing when I was being taught how to suction myself in preparation for my ultimate discharge.

As I recuperated and felt stronger, I kept asking my surgeons about moving me out of the SICU. I felt that getting out was a sign that I was well on my road to recovery. It symbolized to me a sort of "graduation" from the dependent helpless stage to a more independent one. The great day finally came, and I was happy to be moved out. I was hoping to find myself in a quieter and more efficient place where I was to receive more specialized care by a team of nurses with greater expertise in caring specifically for head and neck patients.

Chapter 14. Going to the Regular Floor

After four days in the SICU, I was wheeled out of my cubicle and out of the SICU to an elevator. On my way out, I realized how crowded the SICU was. It looked so different compared to the way it had when I first saw it a few weeks earlier during my tour of the hospital. Previously, it seemed to me like any other SICU I had visited as a guest speaker – just a place to observe and learn about interesting or complex patients. Now I looked at it as one of those patients that was lucky enough to get out of it alive.

The hospital was an awkward assembly of three different buildings, joined together over seven decades into a giant building, filling up two New York City blocks. On a wing of the eighth floor, overlooking Lower Manhattan, the elevator stopped at the Otolaryngology Ward, a specialized unit for Dr. Marker's patients. As Dr. Marker had told me, I ended up first in the Step-Down Unit, which serves as a transitional unit between the SICU and the regular ward. The Step-Down is situated in a large room, with four beds and is staffed by two nurses.

Most of the nurses were very competent and effective. However, there were some who were less experienced and just rotating through. Because it was so small, the nurses were stationed very close to the patients' beds and could respond almost instantly. Most of the patients stayed in the Step-Down Unit for four to five days until they became more stable and could be moved to the regular ward. When I visited the hospital a few weeks prior and walked through the hallways, I did not notice that unit, where critical recovery happened after the patients were transferred from the SICU.

The care I received there was more personal and efficient, which made me feel better and reduced my discomfort. I wished such care could have been provided when I was much more in need of it during my stay in the SICU.

I was bedridden for most the time in the unit but gradually started to ambulate, especially after I was disconnected from some of the equipment. Getting out of bed was complicated and took some time and assistance. I had to remove the monitoring cables, release myself from the breathing mask that covered my stoma site, secure the intravenous line and fluid bag, and, when the urine catheter was still in, navigate it to a comfortable position.

I spent most of the hours of the day throughout my hospitalization in bed because I was still very tired and restricted by all the lines and instruments that were connected or attached to me. These included intravenous line, monitoring cords, oxygen mask, and catheter. Over time, some of these were removed, but because of my swollen and stiff neck, I could not lie down or sleep on any side except my back, which became difficult after a while. I started to sit up on a chair by my bed and spent several hours a day there, even becoming able to fall asleep in this position. I began listening to my favorite stations on the radio, which helped me get connected to the outside world again.

One of the first roadblocks I had to overcome was to teach myself to stand up again. It was more difficult than I had expected. I wanted to do that so that I could go to the bathroom by myself. I felt off-balance for a few seconds but was able to steady myself. I was even able to wash myself with a towel in the bathroom after assuring the nurse that I would call for assistance if needed. I began to take short walks in the long corridors of the floor, in the beginning very slowly and carefully always carrying my intravenous fluid bag that was hung over a pole. My son and wife would generally escort me, and I gradually increased the distance I covered and the frequencies of the walks. I was encouraged to take these walks by the nurses because this facilitated my recovery, prevented blood clots from forming in my legs, and decreased the swelling in my neck.

I was able to finally check my email using one of the computers in the family waiting room, which was staffed by a very caring and helpful woman. She was the one who had called me prior to the surgery and was very helpful to my family throughout the hospitalization. A great moment of relief came when the arterial catheter was pulled out and I got rid of one fluid line. Next came the removal of the urine catheter. I was apprehensive to have it pulled out because I was afraid that I would have difficulty passing urine by myself but, happily, this did not occur.

One of the most important tasks that had to be constantly performed on me was to repeatedly suction my trachea to remove accumulated mucus and clean the tracheostomy tube. I could not clear these secretions myself because the tube was a foreign body that had to be physically cleaned. The nurses put on sterile gloves and used a special sterile suctioning kit. They connected a catheter to a tube that suctioned the secretions into a special collection bottle. They often inserted sterile saline into the trachea to moisten the secretions so that they would be more easily removed.

A few times a day, the plastic tracheostomy tube was taken out for cleaning. This included immersing it in a hydrogen peroxide solution, which had to be thoroughly washed out afterwards and the tube scrubbed with a special brush. Eventually, the nurses instructed me and my wife how to perform these procedures so that we could do them after my discharge. Over time, the frequency of suctioning decreased from every two to three hours to once every six hours, twelve hours, and eventually, I did not require them at all. This occurred because my trachea adjusted to the direct inhalation of air and produced fewer secretions; also, I was able to cough out the secretions by myself as I regained my strength.

Even though I depended on suctioning and cleaning, I resented the procedure because it was very annoying and irritating. Each suctioning was started with introducing sterile saline into my trachea, which generated very strenuous and explosive coughing that interfered with my breathing and shot blood to my eyes. When I looked in the mirror during these episodes, I noticed that the blood vessels on my face and forehead stood out when I was coughing so hard.

Some of the patients in the unit were sicker than I was and had undergone a variety of surgeries to their heads and necks. These included surgeries to remove cancers of the tongue, jaw, and throat; most were unable to talk. I remember wheeling my intravenous line next to a room with a bedridden man whose face was swollen. He stared impassively at the television in his room. Every day on the ward, I grew stronger, but this patient stayed the same. I never saw him emerge from his bed. It was a reminder to me of how sick I could have become and how lucky I was to have avoided his fate.

One of the frightening episodes that I experienced during my stay on the unit was the sudden emergence of significant swelling of my neck. Even though I had developed some swelling after the surgery, five days later, I noticed that my neck and chin had significantly increased in size within three to four hours. I could no longer move my neck, and even the bag over my tracheostomy site was squashed by the swelling. I immediately notified the nurse and requested to be seen by the doctor on call. The young resident, who was cross covering the ward with another hospital, examined me and assured me that neck swelling was very common after the type of surgery I had. He explained that it was usually caused by the accumulation of lymphatic fluid that could no longer drain through the lymphatic system, which had been removed. It had built up because the drainage now is slower, and it might take months for the lymphatic to establish an alternative route for drainage.

I explained to him (in writing) that I was concerned by the suddenness and rapidity in which this swelling occurred, especially since it had been five days since the surgery. I would have accepted his explanation if the swelling would have happened just a short time after the surgery. I was afraid that the rapid accumulation of fluid was due to an infection or bleeding. I insisted that he consult with Dr. Marker, who was the attending physician on call. He did so while standing near my bedside and informed me that Dr. Marker agreed with his assessment. I was happy and reassured by the attending's response but requested also that my wife talk to him over the phone. Happily, the doctors were correct. It took six months for the swelling to recede with the help of physical and massage therapies.

The new reality of having no voice struck me at that time. I was unable to express myself fully and could not show my emotions. I had to completely depend on the slow process of writing everything on the board. After switching to writing in a notebook, I was able to communicate with greater ease, partially because I no longer needed to erase what I had written earlier and could write longer sentences. I could prepare a longer list of questions for my doctors, and this actually made the writing of this book easier because I had a written record of all of these events. However, having so many bottled in and unexpressed feelings was difficult. The versatility of altering my voice and showing emotions while speaking was gone. I sometimes tried to communicate with my family by lip speaking simple words without any voice. Getting angry or upset was impossible, and my frustration at my inability to speak made it even more difficult. This created more tension and conflicts with my family.

In retrospect, I regret not using an electro-larynx (or artificial larynx – a handheld vibration-producing device placed in the mouth or over the neck) immediately after my surgery. I learned only after my discharge from members of my local Laryngectomee Club that many of them were able to start speak again a few days after their surgery with the help of this device. I could have obtained an electro-larynx prior to my surgery by either purchasing or borrowing it from the Club. Even though I eventually elected not to use this means of communication and to instead use a tracheal-esophageal prosthesis, having an electro-larynx would have helped me tremendously and made my recovery smoother and easier. I would not have had to rely on writing everything down, and I could have started to communicate with everyone in a more natural way, sparing me the trauma of verbal isolation that lasted over two months. Since none of the other patients on the Otolaryngology Ward used an electro-larynx, I assume that the doctors and speech therapists at that hospital did not want to encourage the use of this device and were afraid that once patients get used to it, they would not explore the use of voice prosthesis. Although prosthesis assisted speech sounds more natural, it can only be used after the site of the surgery has healed.

After four days in the Step-Down Unit, I was transferred to the regular ward. I was initially apprehensive about being moved, as the level of nursing was much less intense in the regular ward. However, I saw it as an essential stage in the process of my recovery. All the post-surgical rooms in the ward were small but had a single bed. This was the first time I had some privacy, although the room's sliding door stayed open most of the time. The nurses worked for twelve-hour shifts and were very experienced in caring for post-surgical patients. However, some were better than others, and over time, I learned their strength and weaknesses. I looked forward to being taken care of by the most efficient and caring ones and resented having to deal with those that were less efficient, indifferent, or had an unfriendly and sometimes rude attitude. The nurses that worked in the evenings and nightshifts were generally less experienced and consequently provided less effective care and made more mistakes.

I started to resent the repeated interruptions of my sleep by nurses who took my blood pressure and pulse in the middle of the night or insisted on drawing blood at five a.m. I requested that these night-time checkups be reduced to a minimum. What also was very annoying was the occasional inconsiderate behavior of some of the nightshift personnel who would talk very loudly and on occasion even shout to each other in the corridor outside my room, disregarding the fact that they may wake up resting patients who had probably struggled to get to sleep in the first place. On one occasion, two nurses were arguing with each other. They got so angry at each other that they were shouting for over ten minutes with complete disregard to the sleeping patients around them. It was almost like a street fight between individuals who were night guards in a graveyard, carelessly assuming that no one could hear them. This pattern of behavior was very disturbing and inconsiderate and had not stopped even after I confronted the nurses.

I observed that for some employees, the hospital was just a workplace, but the best caregivers considered it a special place for healing and recovery. Their attitude transmitted through their patient care and improved my recovery.

Throughout my hospitalization, I repeatedly inquired about the pathological results of the specimens taken from the removed tumor. Dr. Marker kept telling me that these were not yet available and it would take some more time for the results to come back. In light of my experiences after the previous surgeries, I was eager to get the results.

My family was very supportive of me and, as before, I was never left alone from about nine a.m. to ten p.m. I had to literally urge my wife to leave the hospital and get some breaks throughout the day, especially when one of my children came. Unfortunately, by the time my wife arrived in the morning, the senior surgeon had already made rounds, and she could not get any direct information from him and relied only on my written reports. My daughters would come after work, and my son visited several times throughout the day. Even though I was looking forward to these visits, it was taxing and tiring at times, especially in the evenings when my small room was full of visitors and friends.

As I was improving, I started to feel the need to rest and be left on my own. Even though the visitors were well intentioned, it occasionally became cumbersome for me. I assumed that they could not appreciate how tired and worn out I was. I was too embarrassed to tell them how difficult it was for me to entertain so many people at one time, but eventfully, I shared this with my wife. I had to urge them almost every evening to go home about nine p.m. and actually started to look forward to finally be left alone so that I could rest. I understood for the first time why hospitals used to restrict and limit guests' visits.

Even still, my family members assisted me and were instrumental on numerous occasions in making sure that I was getting cared for. They reminded or requested staff members to perform different tasks they had neglected or were slow in performing and ensuring that these were carried out. They also prevented errors and reported them. It was so essential for me to get this help, as I was voiceless and bedridden throughout most of my hospital stay.

Although the medical care I received in the ward was overall very good, I realized that mistakes were being made at all levels of my care. Fortunately, I was able to prevent many of them, but not all.

Some of the mistakes made by nurses and other staff members included not cleaning or washing their hands and not using gloves when indicated, attempting to deliver viscous medications through the feeding tube (which clogged the tube), forgetting to connect the CALL button when I was bedridden and unable to speak, and forgetting to write down verbal orders.

One instance that was stressful and hazardous occurred at about five p.m. when the nurse did not respond to my call to suction my airways. I felt difficulty in breathing, as mucus which had built up in my trachea was obstructing my airway. I pressed the CALL button in my room, but no one came to my assistance. I was bedridden, and getting out of my bed was very difficult, as I needed to carry with me the intravenous line and disconnect the tube that delivered oxygen. After repeatedly calling for assistance without any response, I was able to get the attention of a nurse assistant who was not trained in suctioning airways but promised to look for a nurse who could help me. She came back and told me that my nurse was on an hour break and then left my room.

After waiting for some time, I got out of my hospital bed and found another nurse assistant and asked her to get me help. She returned shortly and informed me that she told an RN about my needs, but that nurse was on the phone ordering supplies. Another nurse finally responded, but she could not find any saline solution container, which is needed to rinse the trachea. Finally, the nurse who was on the phone came and performed the suctioning and changed my clogged tracheostomy inner tube. This was a very distressing event as I was agitated and struggling to breathe in the middle of the Otolaryngology Ward. There were two residents and several nurse assistants in the floor, yet no one helped me for what felt like a very long time, although the delay took only about fifteen minutes. I brought the incident to the attention of the nurse supervisor but never received any feedback from her about what would be done to prevent such incidents in the future. My concern was that even on a ward dedicated to people with breathing difficulties and breathing issues, there were many distractions that prevented physicians and nurses from paying attention to their patient's immediate needs.

The most serious error was prematurely feeding me by mouth with soft food. This happened eight days after my surgery when the speech therapist whom I had not met before walked into my room about four p.m. and informed me that I could start eating food through my mouth. I was surprised, because I remembered that Dr. Marker had told me when I first saw him that I would not be able to eat anything by mouth for about two weeks. This was because the flap had to be integrated into the esophagus, and the post-surgical swelling needed to come down before I could resume eating. Although I was happy to hear that I was well enough for the doctors to allow me to eat by mouth, I wrote down my concerns for the speech therapist to see, but she assured me that this was approved by the physicians.

She proceeded to feed me with small amounts of dyed liquid to see if the food leaked from anywhere around my neck. After no leak was observed, she proceeded to feed me small amounts of jello and applesauce. I was very happy to be able to eat again but still felt unsure whether this was really allowed. I called for the resident, and he confirmed that it was okay for me to start eating. I received a liquid dinner and ate about half of it. I felt too full to eat all the food and preferred to continue receiving formula through my feeding tube.

I kept worrying about eating so soon after the surgery, and when the senior attending made his morning rounds sixteen hours later, I asked him if it was safe for me to eat. He acted bewildered when he heard that I was allowed to eat and ordered it stopped right away. Fortunately, I had not yet received my breakfast. Eventually, I was allowed to resume eating by mouth only a week later. I was very upset and worried about the consequences from eating prematurely. I worried that this would interfere with the healing of the sutures inside my neck and lead to failure of the flap to integrate. Fortunately, this did not happen, although ten days later, I experienced a leakage of fluid from the flap into the neck, although, I was not sure if this was because of the premature exposure to food. I was fortunate to have persisted in questioning the logic of allowing me to eat. This serious error occurred because of miscommunication of verbal orders between the residents who wrote an order to start feeding another patient on my chart instead of the other patient's chart.

All of these events made me wonder what happens to patients without medical education who cannot recognize and prevent an error. Since recent studies had shown that medical errors occur in up to 40 percent of patients hospitalized for surgery and up to 18 percent of them suffer from complications because of these errors, I should not have been surprised. However, it was difficult to experience these mistakes myself. I also wondered what would have happened if I would not have continued to question the feeding and when (or if) the error would have been eventually discovered. Fortunately, despite these errors, I did not suffer any long-term consequences. However, I had to be constantly on guard and stay vigilant, which was very exhausting, especially during the difficult recovery process.

After about twelve days of hospitalization, I began to feel an increasing urge to leave the hospital. I could no longer bear being woken up at night, lying on my back all the time, unable to sleep while turning my head to either side, getting blood drawn, have an intravenous needles stuck in my arm, watching over the nurses to be sure they were not making errors, and the dependency on others. I strongly felt that I had enough. I was looking forward to finally be discharged.

I was eventually allowed to gradually start eating by mouth on the fourteenth day of hospitalization. In the beginning, I was given only liquids, and within two days, I was able to consume soft foods. These changes were coordinated with a proportionate reduction in the tube feedings. Eating by mouth was a relief but was associated with some difficulties. It took me three hours to eat a meal, as I had trouble swallowing the food and needed to mix it with water in my mouth and constantly drink liquids to flush it down. I could not ingest large amounts of food, as my stomach had probably shrunk. I also sensed pressure and pain in my stomach after I ate which was only relieved by burping the air I had swallowed. Unfortunately, burping became very difficult and took a lot of effort, but that ability improved after a few days.

An indication of how much I missed eating by mouth was that I had recurrent dreams about eating regular food and experienced worries that I was doing something wrong. I have never dreamed about eating before, but not getting any food by mouth made this a desired and forbidden quest. Being allowed to resume eating was a sign that my discharge home was imminent.

In preparation for discharge from the hospital, the nurses instructed me and my wife about suctioning the trachea and cleaning the tracheostomy tube. We had several nurses explain this to us, and each of them presented a different method, which was very confusing for us. What was critical in the eyes of one nurse was not even mentioned by another. To add to the confusion, we observed the speech pathologist and the residents performing a completely different cleaning procedure than the nurses did, which was much less strict and opened a window for contamination of the airways because they did not use sterile techniques and rinsed and cleaned the tracheostomy tube with mere tap water.

Before leaving the hospital, I was visited by a social worker who made sure I had the supplies and equipment necessary for maintaining my tracheostomy sent to my daughter's apartment where I planned to stay for a week. I was told that it was mandatory for me to rent a suction machine, even though I had not needed to be suctioned at all for the past two days because I was able to clear my secretions myself by coughing.

I had a list of questions for the doctors that originated from my fear of being away from immediate medical attention and the need to perform many of the tasks carried by experienced medical personnel myself. "Are there any limitations on lifting or moving heavy objects? How do I shower without getting water into my trachea?

Will my neck sensation come back? Can I travel back to Washington DC in a car without breathing humidified air? How do I deal with an emergency situation and can I get help if I need it? Can I be left alone? How do I continue to care for my hand and thigh wounds? And how do I prevent swallowing air when eating, which causes the uncomfortable pressure in my stomach and the need to burp?" They had answers for some of my questions, but not all of them.

I was happy to finally leave the hospital after fifteen days of hospitalization. On my way out, I had to stop at the Otolaryngology Clinic several blocks away. The nurses suggested that I take a taxi to ease my transition back into the normal world and prevent any trauma to my wounds. However, I elected to walk over there rather than be driven. It was important for me to test my independence and walk on my own outside the hospital. It was very strange and disorienting to be in the street again and breathe regular air rather than humidified oxygen. I was worried that I could not accomplish it but, happily, the short walk was not too difficult.

At the clinic, I was seen by the SLP whom I had met before at that clinic and she removed the feeding tube that was inserted through a hole into my trachea and from there reached the esophagus. She replaced it with a voice prosthesis through the same hole and asked me to produce some sounds. I was barely successful and only able to utter a few sounds by sealing my stoma with my thumb. I was afraid that I would never be able to speak again and the prosthesis placed in my neck would not enable me to utter a word. It was difficult and frustrating to try to speak, mostly because the stoma was too large, and I could not cover it completely with my finger. However, the SLP was very supportive and assured me that I would eventually be able to produce a voice that would become audible. She instructed me how to care for my airways by using a humidifier and suctioning and inserted a new tracheostomy tube that did not have an inner tube and was easier to care for. She told me that I would need to breathe through the tube for about a month to insure that the opening of the trachea (stoma) would not shrink after more healing occurred. The SLP was confident, patient, and experienced and spent a long time with me and my family. Even though I had met with her prior to the surgery, only now was I able to appreciate how helpful she really was.

Although I was disappointed that I could not speak yet, I met another patient on my way out of the clinic. He was a butcher who had a laryngectomy a year earlier. His voice was scratchy but self-assured, and he had an unmistakable Brooklyn accent. Meeting him after my first failed attempt to speak gave me some hope that eventually I would be able to communicate as he did.

I was breathing now through a short tracheostomy tube that was covered by a newly installed heat and moisture exchanger (HME) filter. The HME acted as a filter but also increased the humidity within my lungs. I was given another appointment in a week to return to be examined by Dr. Marker and the SLP, after which I was hoping to be able to return to Washington DC. I was still apprehensive about being on my own, but I was reassured that if any problem should occur, there was always a senior surgeon on call.

A few hours after arriving at my daughter's home, boxes of supplies arrived, as did the suction machine later in the evening. We found out that the packages I received were missing several important items, and my wife had to repeatedly call the supply company to get these. The suction machine was brought only after the technician called three times to inform us that she was running late. When she finally arrived at nine p.m., we found her to be impatient, unfriendly, and abrasive. Initially, I tried to explain to her that I did not need or want the suction machine, but she brushed me off, informing me that the hospital regulations required that I go home with it. She briefly explained how to operate the machine, and I was happy to see her leave. I never used that machine but having it gave me some measure of security. We returned the suction machine about a month later, but the rental company kept charging Medicare for more than a year in spite of my protests.

I was apprehensive about meeting my five-year-old granddaughter, who had not seen me after the surgery. I hoped that she would understand that I could not speak and had a tracheostomy tube covered by the HME. I was surprised and happy that she had no trouble adjusting to the way I looked and accepted me as I was without any problems. What might have helped was that I had told her prior to my hospitalization that I would be having surgery, and my daughter had prepared her for my discharge by explaining my condition. I discovered that children can quickly adjust to new realities with fewer difficulties than adults.

It was strange to spend the first night outside the hospital. Even though I was hospitalized for only fifteen days, it felt much longer, and my life had changed so much during that period. I suddenly had to take care of my needs myself, including preparing my food, cleaning my tracheostomy tube and trachea, taking the medications accurately, and caring for my wounds. I slept in my granddaughter's small room that became completely engulfed by the steams produced by the vaporizer. I set all the supplies and added more lights to the small bathroom, which became the center for caring of my stoma. Cleaning the tracheostomy tube was labor-intensive, and I used the supplies I received for this.

I continued to eat by mouth, although it was still difficult. The food kept getting stuck in my throat, and the burping and pressure in my stomach lasted up to two hours after each meal. I had no control of the burping, and when it came, I felt embarrassed and frequently apologized. Even though I had asked for help from several of the surgical attending and the SLP how to deal with this problem, they had no advice for me and just ignored my questions. I sent an email to Dr. Marker asking his input but received no response. Happily, this problem resolved spontaneously within three days.

I spent almost all my days in the apartment but with the encouragement of my family was able to take short walks with them in the neighborhood. I was worried, however, about breathing the outside non-humidified dusty city air and exposure to car fumes. I also felt quite tired and wondered if I had low levels of thyroid hormone because half of my thyroid gland had been removed during my recent surgery.

Unfortunately, an unexpected complication occurred three days after my discharge. About five p.m. on Saturday, I noticed local bleeding, which spontaneous emerged from a site in the right side of my neck on the border between the normal skin and the round bulky bump that was created to check for the flap viability. After drinking warm soup, I noted warm fluid coming out of my neck at the site that had previously bled. When I tried to drink water, I observed clear fluid coming out of a tiny hole in my neck. I was very concerned because it suggested that an abnormal connection has formed between my upper airways and the skin (called a fistula). I was previously told about this potential complication and was wondering if it had actually happened to me. I took my temperature and pulse rate, and both were slightly elevated, suggesting that an infection might have developed at the fistula site.

I asked my wife to call the phone service of the surgeon on call for the hospital and requested to have Dr. Marker paged so that he could contact us as soon as possible. I also sent him an email. After an hour had passed and he had not returned a call (in spite of two reminder calls to the phone service), I requested that they call another attending physician. Happily, that physician responded within twenty minutes and informed us that Dr. Marker was out of town and that he was the surgeon on call. I wondered why the phone service had not known about it. He agreed with me that I had most likely developed a fistula and asked that I return to hospital as soon as possible and go directly to the emergency room. He promised to make sure that the resident on call would expect me. When I requested my wife to ask him what would be done to care for this condition, he brushed me off by stating, "You will soon find out." I was left with an uncertain feeling, but I had no time to waste to ponder it. My short vacation from the hospital had ended abruptly, and I was on my way back again for uncertain times.

Chapter 15. Returning to the Hospital

I arrived in the Emergency Room knowing that what waited for me was readmission to care for the complication that just occurred. The fistula that had been formed was a post-surgical connection that had developed between the inside of my lower throat and the skin in my neck. I expected that I would not be able to eat by mouth for a while to allow the fistula to close and also to receive antibiotics to combat the local infection that had developed. I was hoping that the fistula that had just burst open would heal rapidly and that this would not reverse my recovery. Although my doctors had previously informed me that a leaking fistula could occur in up to ten percent of patients after this kind of surgery, I had hoped, of course, that it would not actually happen to me. I wondered if the fistula developed in my case because of the premature feeding that I had received several days earlier, but there was no way to prove that.

Returning to the hospital was disappointing but necessary. It was Saturday evening, and the emergency room was crowded to capacity. Strangely, I felt comfortable in the emergency room, probably because I had spent a lot of time in this setting before. I worked in the emergency room as a nurse during the two last years of my medical schooling, as a physician in training and also moonlighted in emergency rooms as a physician for more than six years. I had learned from those experiences to stay very calm and focused and perform well in a crisis situation. However, this was different – I was not managing a crisis but was a patient with one. It was difficult to stay calm, but being in the hospital made me feel more secure that my problem would be taken care of. Fortunately, as a returning patient who was expected to be readmitted, the waiting time was brief. It was an old-style emergency room made of a single large hall separated by curtained partitions where individual patients were lying on their gurneys. There was only a small space for each cubicle, allowing for only minimal privacy, and there was no room for any chairs at the patients' bedside for family or friends to sit.

Despite the commotion, I was processed within a relatively short period of time, and after about half an hour, the resident physician and a senior resident on call examined me. They had me drink water with methylene blue color. Several seconds later, a few drops of the colored water emerged on my neck skin, which confirmed that I had indeed developed a fistula. They told me that it was good that I had stopped eating and had come to the hospital right away so that the fistula would not grow larger. They acknowledged that I would definitely receive antibiotics, would not be allowed to eat food by mouth, and would have to stay in the hospital for about two weeks until my fistula closed. They removed the voice prosthesis and replaced it with a feeding tube, returning me to the situation I had been in only three days earlier. They also placed a tube in my neck through the incision site to drain any accumulated fluids. Blood was drawn, an intravenous fluid was started, and I was wheeled up to the Otolaryngology Ward that I knew so well. I was hoping that this re-hospitalization would be easier for me because I generally felt stronger and was familiar with the hospital routines.

In the ward, I was given a different room just across the corridor from my previous one. I met again the same familiar nurses and patients, and it felt like I was back in after a short vacation in the outside world. I soon realized than even though I had given my admitting doctor the exact list of medications and their dosages, there were some that were missing in his orders and still others had been prescribed at a different dose. *Why is it so difficult to get it right?* I wondered. *Why did they not look up my older medical or pharmacy records?*

An important difference in my general care was that I no longer needed intermittent suctioning of my trachea because the amount of secretions I produced was reduced. This was a great relief for me, because the process was very irritating and often had to be done rapidly to avoid an obstruction. However, my tracheostomy tube still needed cleaning two or three times a day. I came up with a way to clean my trachea and remove the secretions and mucus by preemptively removing them with a swab. This reduced my urge to cough and my dependence on repeated suctioning.

The special bandages that were placed on the skin donor site on my left thigh, as well as on the flap retrieval site on my left arm, needed to be replaced at least once a day. Unfortunately, the thigh bandage became filled with serous secretion, broke up frequently and also needed at least daily changing. Preventing the breaking of the dressing was difficult because contact with my bed sheets or clothes often damaged the delicate plastic cover, leading to leakage.

I came up with a simple improvisation that shielded the wound site from contact with objects and extended the life of the dressing. I used an empty intravenous line kit box to cover the wound and taped it to the skin. This worked very well in preventing inadvertent damage to the cover, especially while I was asleep. The surgeons liked the idea and complimented me on it. They even suggest that I patent it, so I asked my son to take a picture of it, and a few months later, I submitted my idea in a form of a short manuscript to the "Technical Ideas" section in an otolaryngology journal where it was published for other physicians to see. I had often come up with simple improvisations because I grew up in a period of shortages, rationing and lack of many devices. If something did not work or there was a need for a quick fix for a problem, I came up with a solution.

As I had done in previous hospitalizations, I needed to watch the nurses – especially those on the nightshift – to make sure that they performed the procedures correctly. I observed a serious breach of the standards of care almost daily. Although the general care was adequate, it was very disappointing for me to observe sporadic poor quality of delivery of basic medicine. I always informed the staff when they made a mistake, but on many occasions, it was only after I had been exposed to the errors. Several nurses did not put on gloves to handle me or the instruments that were attached to me, and some came into my room wearing gloves they had used in other rooms. This is a setup for transferring bacteria from patient to patient. On one occasion, the nurse drew my blood after trying three times and then sent it for the incorrect test. I had to have blood drawn again for that test.

My tracheostomy tube had to be cleaned from mucus every eight to twelve hours, which involved a strict procedure using a sterile kit and sterile water. However, several nurses (and, on one occasion, a resident physician) rinsed the tube with non-sterile tap water rather than sterile solution. Several nurses did not rinse away the hydrogen peroxide used for cleaning the tracheal breathing tube, thus causing severe irritation to my trachea, and one nurse connected the suction machine directly into the suction port in the wall, bypassing the special collecting bottle. By doing this incorrectly, she allowed my secretions to contaminate the hospital tubing system. One medical technician took my temperature without placing the thermometer in a plastic sheath, exposing my mouth to potentially harmful bacteria. Even though I was not supposed to eat anything by mouth, on two occasions, I was brought a tray of regular food by a food handler.

Only twice during my hospitalization did a nurse or doctor listen to my heart and lungs or inspect any part of my body except the wounds. In this, I realized that a most basic and essential component of patient care of examining a patient was missing. Doctors nowadays are relying on sophisticated tests such as MRI and CT scans rather than making a diagnosis by examining the patient. Although all medical students are still taught how to examine patients, head and neck surgeons apparently rarely perform these examinations once they have begun their practice.

When I eventually started to receive antibiotics through my feeding tube, I faced another set of problems in ensuring that the nurses did it correctly. Rather than administering a pediatric suspension (which would have easily gone down through the narrow feeding tube), the pharmacy sent two large tablets at each administration time that had to be crushed down and dissolved in water. Unfortunately, the tablets did not dissolve well, and the material had to be constantly shaken to maximize solubility. Many nurses did not shake the solution repeatedly; consequently, the medication did not go through the tube. One nurse used very hot water to dissolve the powder. I was not aware of it at first and only realized that she had done it when I felt the burning pain created by the hot water as the fluid went down my esophagus. I stopped her from continuing by blocking her hand when she tried to push the medicine into the tube, and I had to explain in writing that "Hot water hurts and may cause burn injury to my TEP site, esophagus, and stomach!" Furthermore, I knew the heat could destroy the potency of the antibiotic, rendering it useless. I insisted that she get new tablets from the pharmacy and dissolve and administer them properly, which she begrudgingly did.

I requested that the nurse supervisor and resident physician were informed about this inappropriate mode of dissolving medication so that it was not used with other patients. I was disappointed to see that the resident was not impressed by what I told him, and I did not sense that he was going to do anything with the information. This was an example of how I was able to abort and avoid the harmful effects of an inappropriate practice. I was fortunate to recognize this as a physician and wondered again how patients without medical backgrounds could protect themselves.

Another set of difficulties I had was insuring that the antibiotic was delivered with food, as is indicated in the medication package insert. This timing was needed to reduce the risk of antibiotic-associated diarrhea. Unfortunately, the antibiotic was not scheduled to be given that way and it took numerous requests to change the schedule; and even after it was changed, the nurses repeatedly tried to give it to me at the wrong time. I had a similar issue in scheduling the timing of delivery of the thyroid hormone – a drug that had to be given on an empty stomach at least thirty minutes before feeding. It took four days before the nurses got it right and, even then, I had to remind the staff to give it early so as to not interfere with the feeding schedule.

I also had to constantly remind the nurses to flush my feeding tube with water after each feeding to prevent it from being clogged. If that would have occurred, the tube would have had to be replaced, which would be an elaborate and painful procedure. Since they often neglected to do that, I eventually did it myself. I also learned to control my liquid feedings myself by starting them when I actually felt hungry and slowing their rate or pausing them when I felt full.

I had to repeatedly remind the nurses not to take my blood pressure from my left arm because my flap had been removed from that arm it was missing several blood vessels. I had also to remind them to temporarily stop the intravenous fluids from flowing into the right arm while taking the measurements. This was to prevent the vein used for the infusion from blowing out.

As my peripheral veins were repeatedly used to draw blood and to insert intravenous lines, there were less of them that were still available. I asked the doctors to minimize the laboratory tests and switch my intravenous antibiotics to oral ones. I also became more assertive in making sure that only experienced personnel drew my blood or started an intravenous line. Initially, it was difficult for me to do that because I did not want to offend anyone, but I realized that I needed to if I wanted to save my veins and avoid pain. I allowed nurses to stick me only one more time after one failure and then requested that someone else try. There was one nurse who repeatedly missed my veins, and I eventually politely asked her to let someone else draw my blood. Dealing with all of these human errors required a lot of effort and consumed the little energy I had, interfering with my ability to relax and rest.

While I was back in the hospital yet again, my family was ready to return to normal life. It was difficult for my family to always appreciate how challenging it was going to be for me to return to our previous life. There was a disconnect between the two worlds that I had to face. About a day after my readmission, my wife told me that my oldest daughter wanted to come from California and celebrate Passover in our house. I had hard time explaining to my wife how premature it was to make such plans, as it might be difficult for me to have many guests because of my general weakness. I had to impress upon her why my present health overrode other issues. I assume it was hard for her to place herself in my shoes and understand how different things were for me. Frustration and anger overcame me on numerous occasions because of my inability to express myself adequately without a voice, and I grew tired of relying only on paper and pen.

As before, I encouraged my wife to leave the hospital and do other things during the day, because I realized that sitting by my side for many hours was taking its toll on her. I also urged her to return to Washington and attend to her work, because she had been away from her office for quite a long time. I told her that things were stable, and the only reason I was in the hospital was to get antibiotics and tube feeding. I assured her that even though she would be away, I would not be entirely by myself because my children would visit me daily. I was afraid that staying in the hospital for such an extended period of time would adversely affect her and felt that she needed a break from everything. Eventually, she consented and left for a few days. Even though I missed her, I felt that this was the right thing to do.

As in my previous hospitalization, it was difficult for me to entertain numerous visitors at the same time. Often, my daughters would come in the evening after eight p.m., which was quite tiring for me. Because I did not want to insult them, I never told them that it was exhausting me, but I encouraged them to go home at around nine-thirty p.m. I think it is often difficult for friends and family to truly appreciate the strain their visits may impose on a hospitalized individual.

I was feeling increasingly tired and assumed that this was the result of the local infection caused by the fistula or perhaps a side effect of the antibiotics I was getting. A lower thyroid hormone level in my body could have also been responsible. I was already receiving replacement thyroid hormone because of the moderate hypothyroidism I developed after the radiation treatment. However, the removal of half of my thyroid gland during my recent surgery most likely increased my need for replacement. I knew that even though my need for replacement hormone would increase, it would take a few weeks for this to become apparent, because the body has stores of the hormone. I repeatedly asked my surgeons to order a blood test to measure my thyroid functions, and they finally did so two days before my discharge. My suspicions were correct, and the hormone levels were indeed low. They increased the hormone replacement dose, but since the body response to the increase is always delayed, it was weeks before I became more energetic and less worn out.

For the first time in weeks, I was able to read a book and listen more often to the radio my son bought me. I enjoyed hearing the news and classical music. I also watched a new television series on my laptop on Digital Versatile Discs (DVDs) my daughter and son gave me. A friend of my son who came to visit me brought me a DVD of a movie that had several disturbing scenes. One ridiculed a hospitalized patient after laryngectomy and his inability to speak coherently with an electro-larynx, and another showing the dead body and funeral of a cancer patient. This movie that showed the hopelessness of cancer was definitely an insensitive and poor choice for me, as it was quite upsetting to watch. My son's friend apologized later, admitting he had forgotten that the movie had those scenes.

I finally decided to shave and cut my hair for the first time in over four weeks. Since I had lost sensation in both of my lower checks and neck, I cut myself with a razor and had to use an electric shaver. My son trimmed my hair and did a very good job.

I was able to use the computer in the family waiting room on the floor more frequently to check my email messages and interact with the world again. I even got back to resuming my work. I reviewed several manuscripts about infectious diseases that were sent to me by medical journals. Unfortunately, the family room was often closed after about five p.m. One evening, I found the room door open and went in to use the computer. After a few minutes, a nurse supervisor angrily walked into the room and demanded that I vacate it immediately or she would call security. I tried to explain to her that the door was open, as was often the case in the evenings, and that on several occasions in the past, it had been opened for me by the residents, but she became even more hostile. I wanted to seek help and complain about her inconsiderate behavior but got nowhere – mainly because of my inability to speak or use the phone.

As I was getting better, I started to reflect on my experiences and what I had undergone in the past three weeks. It was definitely one of the most difficult periods in my life. I understood again why some patients elected to give up and ask that no heroic measures be taken to extend their lives. There is a point where the suffering is not worth the benefit of continuing to live. I never arrived at such a conclusion during my previous hospitalizations, but I understood how people could come to such a difficult decision. This was a new revelation for me, as I always fought very hard to save and extend patients' lives, even when they had poor prognosis. What helped me endure the difficult periods and rise back from the depth of hopelessness was my wish to set an example for my children of how to deal with adversity – that one should not give up at difficult times. I also felt a strong belief in life itself and wanted to keep fighting for it.

As had happened during my previous hospitalizations, I became more impatient about staying in the hospital and anxiously wanted to leave the confines of the Otolaryngology Ward. I did not expect to have such a long stay just because of the fistula. I had rarely been hospitalized before the cancer, and my past hospital stays were very short because my recovery was always fast. Even though I was warned and knew that complications may occur, it was difficult to stay so long.

The lack of privacy, the repeated blood drawings, and the sometimes inconsiderate behavior of the staff became more and more annoying. Once, when I requested a nurse, no nurse came to my room from eleven p.m. to five a.m. I was frequently woken up by noisy staff members who ignored the patients' need to sleep by conducting noisy discussions and even shouted loudly in the corridor. The only reason I had to stay in the hospital was to receive tube feeding while my fistula was closing, a process that would take ten to twelve days. I brought this up to my doctors, suggesting that I continue oral feeding at home, and they, in fact, considered it.

A week after my admission, the surgeons took off the dressing that covered the flap site on my left arm. They wanted the area to heal by exposure to air and form a scab. The area hurt intensely for a few hours, but the pain eventually receded.

Nine days after my admission, the doctors decided that it was time to see if my fistula had sealed. To find out if the fistula had stopped leaking, a dye swallow test was performed by a resident. He asked me to swallow a teaspoonful of diluted blue dye and told me to watch and see if blue color appeared on my neck skin at the fistula exit site within an hour of ingestion. I was happy to observe that no blue color appeared on my skin, indicating that healing had taken place. To ensure that the fistula was indeed closed, I was also sent to have a contrast material swallow that was done under X-ray. The radiology resident's initial interpretation was that there was still a leak, but after he showed the study to the senior radiologist, they concluded that there was no leakage.

I started again to receive liquid food by mouth while the amount of the formula I received through the gastric tube was reduced. It was a relief to finally resume eating by mouth, although the quantity of food I ingested was very small in the beginning, and I had to eat very slowly and burp frequently. Because of this, I had to continuously eat throughout the day.

My elation about finally eating by mouth (and therefore expecting to finally leave the hospital) ended abruptly when a few hours later, while I was eating lunch in my hospital bed, I noticed that I was leaking liquid again through the same location in my neck as I did before. Obviously, the fistula had not closed yet. I realized then that the leak occurred only when I swallowed a large amount of liquid, therefore generating more pressure on the liquid to go down my esophagus, which was apparently enough to push it through the fistula. I had to stop eating by mouth, resume formula feeding, and wait longer for the fistula to heal. The food service kept bringing me meal trays to eat for two more days, adding to my frustration. I was so eager to exit the hospital that I considered again the option of leaving and letting the healing occur at home. The reopening of the fistula was a great disappointment for me, as I was ready and eager to leave. But in the greater scheme of things, it was only a minor setback on the road to recovery. The surgeons reassured me that since my fistula was small, it would probably heal in a few more days.

I tried to understand why the methylene blue color swallow test showed no leakage and led to an incorrectly conclusion that the fistula had sealed. When I discussed this with a senior resident, I realized that the test was performed incorrectly. I was given a cup of dyed water and told by the resident to swallow it at my own pace. He left the room but did not instruct me how I should swallow. I cautiously and slowly took very small sips of water because I was afraid to damage anything. If I had swallowed large gulps of water, the leakage would have been evident right away. This was something I remembered when the test was repeated a few days later.

Five days later, the surgeons repeated the dye swallow test, and this time I performed it as it should be done by quickly swallowing large amounts of fluid. Happily, there was no leakage, and I was started again on clear fluids. This time, I was able to eat and drink without any recurrence of leakage. That meant that I was finally on my way out of the hospital and could be discharged the next day.

One day before my discharge, Dr. Marker finally informed me about the pathological report that described the results of the analysis of the tissues removed at the surgery. All the removed lymph glands had no cancer invasion, but there was a very small amount of tumor found around the area where the surgeons in Washington had operated. It took the pathologists over three weeks to come out with the final report. Apparently, their first assessment was that there was no cancer to be found, but the surgeon insisted that they look hard again. Only when they did that two more times did they find a small collection of cancer cells. Apparently, most of the cancer had been removed by the surgeons in Washington, but even a small number of cells would have eventually grown in number and led to recurrence.

To my question "In retrospect, if I had been operated on by an experienced laser surgeon, would I have been able to prevent the need for the extensive surgery?" Dr. Marker reiterated what he had previously told me: the salvage surgery he did was the best one for me from the onset. Having recurrence of cancer after radiation negated, in his opinion, the laser option entirely, and having the total laryngectomy that I had undergone gave me the best chance for cure. It was good to hear him say this again, as I was wondering if what I had endured was actually needed in light of the pathological results.

He further assured me that the entire region where the cancer could grow was removed, and since there were no signs of local or systemic spread, he was very optimistic about my future chances of long-term survival. However, he reminded me that I should be continuously monitored to ensure that there were no recurrences in any other areas of my neck and head and that I should be closely followed throughout my life. The follow-ups should be monthly for the first year after the surgery, every two months the second year, and than incrementally less often.

When the discharge day came, I gathered my belongings as I had previously done and bid goodbye to the residents and nurses. I thanked all of them and hugged the resident who took care of me, expressing my sincere gratitude for all he had done. Even though things were not always perfect, I knew he truly cared for me and did the best he could. As a sign of my gratitude, I gave him a signed copy of the textbook on sinusitis that I authored.

As has been the case two weeks earlier, we stopped at the Otolaryngology Clinic to see the SLP and Dr. Marker. The SLP removed my gastric tube again and inserted a new voice prosthesis in my TEP. I was reinstructed how to take care of my prosthesis, how to clean it by flushing it with water using a small plastic bulb, and how to manually remove the crust and secretions around it. I was also told that as the swelling subsided, the length of the prosthesis would decrease and that, generally, the prosthesis could last for three to six month. The most common problem I might experience would be that liquid might come through the voice prosthesis into my trachea and, if this should happen it should be replaced as soon as possible. To prevent aspiration, the SLP gave me a special plug that could be inserted into the prosthesis until it could be replaced. She also reminded me to squirt small amounts of saline into my trachea a few times a day or when I felt that my airways were dry.

I still had great difficulty verbalizing any word, mostly because I still had a tracheostomy tube inserted in my trachea and could not completely occlude the stoma with my fingers. However, the SLP assured me that I would be able to do that in the future once the neck swelling subsided. She reassured me that I would be able to lecture again, and that there were patients who were able to resume their work as teachers or lawyers after laryngectomy. I asked if I would be able to honor my commitment to give a talk at the Annual Meeting of the American Academy of Otolaryngology on tonsillar infection in five months, and she and Dr. Marker assured me that I could. As they predicted, not only was I able to do that, but I was also able to give my first lecture in ten weeks. However, I decided to excuse myself from giving a lecture scheduled only four weeks later so that the organizers would have sufficient time to find a replacement. I was not sure if I would be ready to speak so soon.

The SLP was an outstanding therapist with extensive experience and resourcefulness. With self-confidence in her approach, she was personally involved with the care of all her patients. She spent extensive amount of time with me and my family and did not let us leave the clinic until I had received complete and thorough treatment.

It was a wonderful feeling to finally leave the hospital. I was hoping not to return there again – or at least not so soon. We returned to my daughter's apartment where I slowly adjusted to life outside the hospital. I resumed taking care of my tracheostomy tube, stoma, and hand wound. I had to clean the tube several times a day using the cleaning kits I received and used the methods the nurses had taught me. I breathed humidified air and had to make sure that my trachea stayed free of secretions.

Even though I was still tired and quite exhausted, I went out on short walks. It was a difficult task to walk even a few city blocks, but my wife and children encouraged me to continue. I was apprehensive inhaling the polluted city air and tried to avoid the busiest streets. I slowly increased my food intake but had to spend a lot of time chewing the food very thoroughly and mixing it with water in my mouth before swallowing. When I forgot to do this, food got stuck in my throat and could only be removed by vigorous manipulation or attempting to vomit. For someone who always finished eating before anyone else, it was quite a change to be the last one to finish his meal.

We returned to the Otolaryngology Clinic two days later for re-examination and further instructions by the SLP. It was reassuring to see that everything was progressing smoothly. The SLP encouraged me to try to talk by covering my stoma with my thumb, thus forcing the expelled air through the prosthesis. The voice that came out was very weak and rusty, and I was still unable to utter many syllables. This was very disappointing, and I was wondering if I would ever be able to speak again. The SLP kept reassuring me that what I uttered then was all that was expected from anyone at this stage of recovery and that my voice would get better over time.

After we left the clinic I decided to try to walk with my wife back to my daughter's apartment forty-five city blocks away rather than take a cab or subway. Surprisingly, I was able to accomplish that feat, although there were times I almost gave up. I had several bouts of intense coughing, but they eventually subsided. I took short rests on the way on city benches and at shops but completed the walk. It took almost two hours, and I felt a great sense of accomplishment at the end knowing that I could return to my old self.

We finally left for home in Washington a day later, partially because I was eager to return home, but also because my granddaughter had developed a cold that I did not want to catch. We decided to rent a car so that we could transport all the medical supplies and equipment I had received. I was apprehensive about being on the road and breathing non-humidified air for several hours and also worried that something would go wrong and I would have difficulty breathing or clearing my airway. I initially suggested to my wife that we take the train, but she insisted that we travel by car so that if any emergency occurred, we could drive to the closest emergency room. I was nervous about renting a car without being able to talk to the rental agent and relying only on writing to do that, but happily, the agent was very cooperative and understanding, which made the process easier.

My wife drove the car, and my son joined us for the ride. He insisted on coming with us so that he could assist us in unloading the car or with anything else we needed. I felt bad that he had to make the long trip with us, but it was comforting to know that he was there in case anything went wrong. After driving for about two hours, I noticed that my wife became very tired and I suggested that I replace her for some time. She initially resisted the idea but consented after a while. I started driving the car, and since my wife and son fell asleep, I continued to drive all the back home. It was actually not difficult to drive, although I had to stop at rest areas to cough and clear my lungs.

It felt great to finally reach home after the month-long ordeal. Ahead lay a long and challenging road of resuming life without my vocal cords – and hopefully, without cancer.

Chapter 16. Surgeons' Attitudes

The attitude of my surgeons was a very important element of my post-surgical care and emotional wellbeing. While the demeanor of the military surgeons in Washington was excellent, my experience was different at the medical center in New York, where the surgeons seemed busier and always in a rush I remain, of course, ever grateful to them for the excellent surgical skills that gave me a second chance for life, but must note that their post-surgical care was less attentive. This difference was probably due to several factors. I had known the surgeons in Washington for some time and worked with some of them before, while in New York, I was new to everyone. In Washington, I was a special case because they did not have a lot of patients with my particular condition; while at the major center for head and neck cancer in New York, I was just one among many – and not even the most serious or complicated case. Also, after I lost my ability to speak after my surgery in New York, responding to my needs and questions required greater amounts of time and patience – something not easily granted by surgeons who are in practice at a for-profit institution. I suspect that they had a heavier patient load and were under greater pressure to perform more surgeries for monetary reason. As the old adage goes, "time is money."

As a physician, I not only wanted to be informed about my condition and treatment, but I also needed detailed explanations of what they were planning to do and why. I also wanted to hear from them all the potential reasons for every condition I had developed, not just the most likely. I needed to have the opportunity to express my opinion and give my input in areas where I was experienced. After recovering from the effects of anesthesia, I was very aware of what was happening to me and was able to report to my caretakers useful input about my symptoms that helped them address issues early on. However, this process became very difficult after I lost my ability to speak and was forced to depend only on writing to communicate.

Surprisingly, the greatest difficulty I had in communication with the staff was with the physicians. I realized that some of my surgeons were impatient, rushing, and always in a hurry to finish rounds, especially when they had surgeries scheduled. I received the attention of the senior surgeons for only a few minutes each day. Rounds were very quick and superficial. The residents would show up early in the morning (around six a.m.), just prior to going to the operating room, and rush through their visits with the patients. Because they were in such a hurry, their visits often consisted of doing nothing more than changing bandages and looking at the surgical wounds. The attending physicians would come at about seven a.m. and would quickly make rounds so that they could also get to the operating rooms or attend their clinics.

A resident physician stayed on the floor all day and performed the ward chores of attending to the wounds and writing orders. However, the resident was often called to assist in the operating rooms, thereby leaving the ward uncovered at times for many hours. This was frustrating for me (and I presume for other patients as well) because any problems or issues that arose went unattended until the floor resident or attending physician's return. Fortunately, in my case, the junior resident was a very friendly and caring individual and did his best to assist and take care of me. When I eventually left the hospital, I told him how grateful I was for everything he did for me and how did his attitude and actions help me recover.

I realized that on many occasions, the residents and attending physicians were making decisions about procedures or changes in medication, and these were never carried out simply because they were failing to write them down. There were occasions when their orders were inscribed a day or more later only after I reminded the doctors about this.

On one occasion, I observed the appearance of new dots in my field of vision which resembled a detachment of the vitreous body in one eye, quite similar to what I had experienced several weeks earlier. I was concerned that my intense coughing would aggravate the condition and potentially even cause a detachment of the retina. I brought this to the attention of the attending physician who told me that he would ask for an ophthalmologist to examine me. The ophthalmologist never came, and I learned that this was because the doctor I spoke with did not fill any consultation request.

One thing I did learn was that it was best for me to prepare a list of questions prior to rounds. Even though I went to the trouble of doing this every day, most of the doctors had very little patience reading these written concerns and would often leave without waiting for me to write down any follow-up questions. When I tried to ask them another question or clarify an issue, they often brushed me off or told me, "Don't worry about it," but this was not enough for me. I wanted to understand why and what was going on, and if I had a new symptom, I needed an explanation of what was causing it and if it was something to be expected in my condition. I felt frustrated by their attitudes.

The highlight of my day was the few minutes I would spend with the doctors as they opened a window into the status of my recovery and complications. I would anxiously wait to see the surgeons each morning. But when the surgical team arrived and departed within two or three minutes without giving me time for follow-up questions, I felt ignored and frustrated. Instead of being an informed partner in my treatment, I felt like a nuisance. I felt that the morning rounds were just an obligation that they did reluctantly – something they wanted to finish as quickly as possible so they could rush to the operating rooms. Sitting alone in my hospital room with so many unanswered questions made me angry. I had no voice to call the physicians back or verbalize my frustration. I was also afraid that if I antagonized them, I would receive even less attention.

The doctors rarely examined any part of my body except for the incisions and flap removal sites and listened to my lungs only when I asked them to do so. The nurses were also inconsistent about listening to my lungs or doing physical examinations. I knew they should have performed more thorough examinations. As otolaryngologists, they limited themselves only to the head and neck and ignored the rest of my body. Medical protocol is that a patient has to be seen and treated as a whole – not as a body system. However, my physicians gave me no time to verbalize my thoughts, and I felt powerless to change their habits.

This was not the medically correct way to care for an elderly patient as I who had major surgery. Medical students are taught the importance of the need for a thorough and complete daily physical examination of each hospitalized patient. This is how I was taught and practiced medicine. As a medical school teacher myself, this is how I instruct future physicians. I assume that physicians nowadays rely more on sophisticated medical tests and less on physical examination. Because of this reliance on technology, I suspect they lose many of their critical examination skills and basic diagnostic abilities. One of the surgeons who reluctantly complied with my request to listen to my heart and lungs jokingly said, "I will do it, but you and I both know that I will not know how to interpret my findings." As much as he tried to make it sound like a joke, I think he was honest and was telling me the truth.

I also encountered abrasive and rude physicians. On one occasion during the early-morning rounds, I asked a senior resident to clean my obstructed tracheotomy tube. He seemed to be very rushed that morning, as the residents always were on days they had surgeries scheduled. This resident had inspected the skin donor site on my thigh and only wrapped it again after I insisted that he complete his work and not leave it open. He reluctantly went on to flush the tracheotomy tube using tap water rather than the sterile cleaning kit and sterile water that were routinely used for this purpose. He did not even use the brush that was included in the cleaning kit, which helps remove the debris. The tube he wanted to place back into my trachea was still dirty, and when I asked him to use the kit and brush the mucus out, he abrasively responded, "We call the shots here," and left my room. His mannerism was condescending, arrogant, and bluntly rude. This was a resident that I had previously noticed to be aloof and condescending, and I never looked forward to seeing him. I felt very humiliated, helpless, and angry after being treated in this fashion. He had shown terrible bedside manners, and his demeanor and behavior were unacceptable.

When I complained about the incident to the attending physician, he did not show any sympathy or understanding. The attending told me that he was surprised at what had happened because that resident had not acted in a similar fashion before, at least not to the best of his knowledge. I never had any follow-up to my complaint. I felt that having no voice and being incapacitated by my recent surgery made it easier for the physicians to ignore me and my feelings. In this case in particular, the surgeons manifested no understanding or sympathy to how a speechless patient feels in being unable to assert himself. In spite of my note to the senior surgeon that said, "It is important to treat a patient – especially one who is unable to speak – with dignity and patience, not to mention showing respect to a colleague," he had nothing to say.

Another disturbing incident occurred on the morning one day before my discharge. A nurse that was tasked to change dressings and bandages removed the special transparent cover that was placed on the denuded skin area on my left thigh. She was inexperienced in the technique and made numerous attempts to replace the bandage. A surgical resident kept correcting and instructing her but left in the middle of the instruction, allowing her to complete the procedure without supervision. After she kept trying to do it and hurting me in the process, I asked her to stop and get the resident to complete the work. She angrily walked out of the room, leaving me in a very uncomfortable position with my wound exposed to the air. After no one came back, I kept calling the nurses for help and asked to page the resident. After about ten minutes, the exposed area became increasingly painful. When I called for a nurse, she offered me Tylenol for the pain, not realizing that what was needed to prevent it was simply to cover the wound again. I kept calling the nurses to request a doctor to come and cover the wound, to no avail. Apparently, the resident that had been in my room before was on call during the previous night; he had left the hospital and therefore did not respond to the pages.

When I saw another resident walk by my room, I waved to him and asked him to cover the wound. He agreed, but before he had a chance to do it, the senior surgeon arrived, and he had to leave and join him for rounds. The surgeon was wearing a winter coat and holding an umbrella, so I assumed he was not planning to spend much time in the ward. When they finally arrived in my room, I handed him the list of questions I had previously prepared. He gave me short answers in a rushed voice, and when I tried to get more detailed answers, he told me, "Have your wife call me in my office to get answers. I need to be in my office now," and walked out of the room to continue the rounds. I did not even have a chance to tell him what had just happened and that I had intense pain in the exposed wound which needed to be covered to stop the pain. Not only did he not notice this on his own but this was a very upsetting and humiliating experience. I had no voice to express my needs, nor the necessary time to express them. He could have ended my misery if he would have allowed me to communicate with him and inform him about my pain. If he would have allowed the resident to cover the wound (which was only a three-minute procedure), my suffering would have ended. The pain was so intense that each minute felt like an hour. I had to wait fifteen more minutes until he finished his rounds before the resident finally covered the wound; just as I had suspected, the pain subsided rapidly after he did it.

Despite all of these misgivings, I am most grateful to all the nurses and physicians who cared for me throughout my hospitalizations and attempted to the best of their abilities to help me. The ultimate surgical removal of my larynx and flap reconstruction was flawless, even though I developed a fistula postoperatively. Most of my caregivers and physicians were compassionate, and I felt their genuine care. Even though some made errors, I am deeply grateful to all of them.

Chapter 17. Recuperation

Finally returning to Washington was a happy occasion, although I was too worn out to be able to fully appreciate it. I was very happy to have my sister and niece visit us from Israel shortly after my return. Unfortunately, I had difficulties speaking at that time, which made it difficult for me to communicate with them. I had to adjust and accept that from then on, I would have to take care of myself without supervision or guidance. I had to clean my tracheostomy site, care for the seal around my stoma site, and make sure that my tracheal secretions were repeatedly cleared. I realized that except for general instructions I received, my doctors and nurses in New York gave me no detailed explanations of how to do that, and even the SLP there only explained about tracheo-esophageal prosthesis care and not about other issues.

I realized that surgeons were not involved with, and some were not even knowledgeable about the basic routine home care after tracheostomy. Most leave it to the SLP, and the ones who cared for me in Washington did not work with me on these issues. I was, therefore, left to my own resourcefulness and improvisations to cope with these tasks. It took me many trial-and-error attempts to come up with ways to actually perform the different tasks.

Even though my surgeon explained to me prior to the operation the procedures I was about to undergo and their consequences, I was not prepared to face the new realities and the difficulties I encountered afterwards. I was unable to digest and internalize these discussions adequately because they were delivered at a time when I was very anxious. I wanted the cancer removed, and at this time, all other issues seemed insignificant. I was unable to imagine how it would feel to lose sensation in large portions of my neck, the ability to smell, and – above all – my ability to speak.

I have had to accept and adjust to life with my new realities and limitations. I continuously remind myself that all of these difficulties and handicaps were worth the chance I have received to beat and survive cancer. Almost every aspect of my life, including regular daily activity, changed. I not only had to adjust to my different voice, but also to the changes in my appearance. I was worried how my wife, friends, colleagues, as well as others would accept me. I was happy to realize that these issues did not pose a major problem, for I was well-accepted all around.

I had a bit of trouble accepting my new self, though. It was overwhelming to face a changed person in the mirror and also face the laundry list of tasks that I had to learn and perform for the first time.

I had to learn to live with fluid reflux into my mouth after bending forward (especially after drinking), difficulty swallowing solid food, the inability to speak while eating, limited motion and loss of sensation in my neck and left arm (because it was a donor site for the flap that reconstructed my larynx), the presence of a "hole" in my neck (my tracheostomy stoma site), swelling of my neck (a neck that now looked different without the Adam's apple), limitation in my head range of motion which created a stiff neck, the constant need to cough and clear my tracheal secretions, the need to spend time several times a day maintaining the cleanliness and patency of the stoma and the tracheo-esophageal prosthesis, waking up about thirty minutes earlier in the morning to devote time to attach the housing for the prosthesis, spending about twenty minutes each night before going to sleep to remove the prosthesis housing and clean the skin around it, the need to order equipment and supplies and always carry these to maintain my airway and stoma, the difficulties in maintaining a seal that enables me to speak using the prosthesis, realizing the fragility of my ability to speak, learning to speak again using the voice prosthesis and all the challenges and technical issues relating to its repeated failures, difficulties being understood while speaking with a weak voice while on the phone and in person, and the discrimination I had to deal with because of my condition. It was a lot to adjust to and was all very physically, emotionally, socially, and mentally demanding.

Upon my return home, I had a growing sensation that I was suffering from a form of post-traumatic stress disorder. I felt that I had just lived through an immensely draining physical and emotional experience where I could not fully express my feelings, was often ignored and sometimes humiliated, and had undergone a major loss of some of my most important capacities and communication skills. I was upset at having to live with so many new handicaps, including my inability to speak adequately. I had frequent anger outbursts, was on the verge of depression, worried constantly, experienced frightening thoughts about my survival and the potential deterioration of my health, avoided people and activities I used to like in the past, had disturbing dreams, and relived many of the horrific events I had recently endured.

Although on the surface I looked and acted more and more like my old self, it was a mere disguise for the benefit of those around me. In reality, I was very tired, partially due to the hypothyroidism that was slow in resolving and partially because of the lingering effects of the surgeries. I wanted to be normal but lacked energy and was constantly disappointed and upset at myself for not being able to frequently go out of the house and join my wife on the weekends. Even going to the theatre or cinema was a challenge because I was afraid that if I needed to cough, my barking sound would disturb others or interfere with the presentation. When I finally did go, I sat in the corner of the theatre so that I could have easy access to the exits in case I needed to leave. To my surprise, I enjoyed going out and never ran out of the theatre in panic.

A simple walk up the hill or just walking in a fast pace became difficult. I experience these difficulties because I can not inhale enough air to meet the requirements of my muscles because the filter that covers my soma limits the amount of air that I can inhale.

My inability to speak at all or only with limited capacity created in me a growing feeling of inner pressure. I felt isolated from the world and from the people around me. Because I had retired from work, I had limited contact with other people, and my main means for communication was through email. Because I could barely speak, I could not use the phone to call others and depended on my wife to take care of things I could not do myself. I also could not express my thoughts and feelings easily and had a buildup of anger and frustration when I could not convey my thoughts and needs. I expected my wife to understand me and read my mind, even though it was impossible for her to do so at all times. This created tension between us, and I had to repeatedly explain and apologize to her for getting angry and frustrated. In retrospect, the experiences we shared together and her devotion and patience to me during the ordeal strengthened our relationship.

What was also very helpful to both my wife and me were the mutual and individual visits to the social worker we had seen before. Initially, it was strange to go to a session and only communicate with the therapist through writing. Her excellent skills, compassion, and understanding were most instrumental in my recovery. We discussed various issues relating to my recovery process, as well as my anxieties and frustrations. She was also helpful on one occasion to straighten out a communication problem I had experienced with my speech therapist.

On one occasion, the social worker began to wonder if I was experiencing depression. I strongly denied this and was even surprised she suggested that I felt that way. However, in retrospect, I realize that she was correct in sensing how difficult it was for me to avoid depression. I was truly struggling with depression lurking inside me, but although there were minutes (and sometimes hours) when I felt depressed, I did not feel permanently so. I was overwhelmed during those times by the multiple tasks I had to perform and the new realities I had to accept. I was mourning the many losses I had experienced, which included my voice, my wellbeing, and the need to accept many permanent deficits. Very early after my return home, I realized that I had a choice to make between succumbing to depression or fighting back and returning to life. I chose the latter because deep inside I had a very strong desire to get better and overcome my handicaps.

I decided to take small steps en route to recovery. One of my first actions was to write to all the colleagues that had responded to my inquiries on how to treat the cancer. I felt great gratitude to all of them, especially since most had never even met me. I updated them about what had transpired during the past three months and thanked them for their support during the challenging period. I ended my message to them with an optimistic tone about my potential good prognosis. Most of them responded by sharing my optimism and wishing me well.

Unfortunately, I had to attend several funerals of my wife's family members in the months following my surgery. I had always found it difficult attending funerals, but this became more difficult after I was diagnosed with cancer because I was more aware and afraid of my own mortality. The first funeral I attended was the most difficult one, and I could not escape the fear that I may be soon the one who would be lying in the coffin. However, I did find meeting family members comforting and enjoyed interacting with them after the actual funeral.

In an effort to break out of the circle of isolation and downhill slide to depression, I started to return to the hospital to participate in medical rounds and listen to medical lectures. Because of my weak voice, I obtained a small microphone so that I could better communicate in crowded places. I tried using it a few times but felt uncomfortable. Eventually, I abandoned its use entirely because my voice became more consistent, and I realized that I can get along without it if the group I was speaking to was small. I noticed that others were listening to me very attentively when I spoke out and were grateful to hear my input. What was most encouraging and rewarding was that my contributions impacted and improved individual patient care. I felt that by going back to the hospital, I was making a difference again. This made me want to return to the hospital and teach even more. In the process of helping others, I was also helping myself.

I was also able to gradually return to many of my other routines. I started with simple challenges such as reading medical literature again, accepting invitations to review articles submitted to medical journals, learning how to take a shower without aspirating water, and even simply walking more. I gradually became able to ride a bicycle and even climb to the top of a small mountain in upstate New York with my family. Even though I realized that the quality of my voice was not the same as before, one of my greatest comebacks was to be able to teach and lecture again with the help of a microphone. Each of these small steps made me feel better and stronger. I was discovering the world again, quite like an infant learning to walk.

Soon after my return home, I started to attend the monthly meetings of the local Laryngectomee Club, as well as their monthly speech therapy sessions. There were about eight regular attendees and several others who came occasionally. Most of them were using an electro-larynx, and a few used a voice prosthesis to speak. I found these meetings very helpful – especially in the first months. The speech therapist was very helpful and had done what my own speech therapists never did: She instructed me on how to speak using my voice prosthesis, gave me very helpful suggestions for its maintenance that helped me overcome many practical problems, and also instructed and encouraged me to use an electrical larynx for the first time. The club president who had met me prior to my surgery lent me an electro-larynx and a microphone, which I returned a few weeks later when I obtained my own set. I used the electro-larynx only until my own voice became stronger, because the sounds it produced sounded too mechanical. However, it served as an excellent substitute, and, in retrospect, I wish I would have had the opportunity to use an electro-larynx earlier during my hospitalization. I was able for the first time to start speaking. I cherished the support and advice I received from the other club members and especially from the club president, who was extremely dedicated and deeply caring and helpful toward the members. I kept coming to the club even when my needs were no longer intense and became its secretary the following year.

One of the most difficult issues I struggled with was the swelling and edema that developed under my chin and in my neck following my surgery, which was compounded by muscle stiffness caused by the radiation I received. These limitations prevented me from moving my head from side to side and attaining a seal around my stoma which was necessary for speech. Furthermore, my left hand (which had a large defect after the skin flap was removed) was weak, and I barely used it. I asked my surgeons in New York whether or not wrapping my neck with an elastic bandage would reduce the swelling, but they discouraged me from doing this because they feared it might interfere with my breathing. However, I eventually decided to wrap my neck with an elastic bandage that I placed very loosely around my chin. I used it only when I went to sleep and was reclining, because when I was awake and upright, gravity enhanced the drainage, rendering the bandage unnecessary. I was amazed by the results, as some of the swelling subsided.

I was fortunate that my surgeon in Washington referred me to a specialist in caring for patients with post-surgical edema and scars at the Breast Care Center in the Navy Hospital. The therapist helped me reduce my neck and left arm swelling, released much of my neck stiffness, and increased my head range of motion. She did it by massaging my swollen areas and stiff muscles and by teaching me exercises that increased their range of motion. Over time, I was able to finally move my head from side to side, which increased my confidence during driving. She had extensive in-depth knowledge in the patho-physiology of post-surgical edema and the recovery processes. She also guided me through the long recovery that gradually increased my ability to function and return to normal activity. Unfortunately, as my Radiation Oncologist reminded me, I needed to keep doing neck exercises throughout my life because irradiated muscles tend to stiffen again. He jokingly called radiation "the gift that continues to give."

After returning home, I was seen by my internist, who performed several blood tests, including measuring the thyroid gland activity. This was done to find out if the increased amount of the thyroid hormone I was receiving corrected the low levels I had. Surprisingly, the tests showed that I had excessive levels and needed to reduce the dose.

After the dose was reduced, repeated measurements done at six- to eight-week intervals showed that the pendulum had swung the other direction, and the levels became lower than desired. Accompanying this decline, I became more tired and lacked energy. The dose was increased again, but this time more gradually and finally the blood levels returned to normal only eight months later.

Ongoing surgeries have had a lasting impact. I had to return to the operating room at the Navy Hospital in Bethesda about eighteen months after my major pharyngo-laryngectomy for a minor orthopedic procedure – the removal of a small cyst from one of my fingers. I had tried valiantly to avoid coming back to the operating room and asked my orthopedic surgeon if she could perform the surgery in the clinic. However, hospital policy required that even small procedures be carried out in the regular operating room. As I expected, returning to the same waiting and surgical rooms was difficult because I had to relive my past painful experiences. I attempted to make myself believe I was only a visitor because my procedure was minimal and required only local anesthesia, but the memories kept coming back. While I was waiting to be taken to the operating room, the head of the Department of Otolaryngology recognized me. He stopped by my gurney to inquire why I was there, and was relieved to learn that I had nothing serious this time.

I did my best to avoid having more surgeries. I was happy to accept Dr Marker's offered to remove the skin tag on the left side of my neck about seven months after my surgery. This tag was part of the tissue that originated from my left hand and replaced my larynx. Having a tag that protruded from my neck allowed the surgeons to monitor the viability of the transplanted tissues after the surgery. However, once it had been established that the transplanted tissues were performing normally, the skin tag, which created a round and unsightly swelling in my neck, was no longer necessary, The procedure to remove the tag was to last only twenty minutes and initially I assumed that it would be carried out in the outpatient clinic. However, a few days prior to the procedure I learned that it had to be done in the hospital operating room. I was reluctant to return to the hospital as a patient because doing so brought back painful memories. However, I decided to go on with the surgery despite my reluctance to return to the hospital.

This was an emotionally difficult task for me. I had to relive the experience of being readmitted, waiting in the pre surgical waiting area, and finally entering the same operating room where I had had my original surgery. Everything around me was familiar but not as ominous as it had been only a few months earlier. Strangely experiencing these conditions again, but under better circumstances, made the process easier and was somehow psychologically therapeutic. This time I was getting surgery for cosmetic reasons and not to save my life. The fact that I was undergoing surgery to look better meant that I had life to look forward to. Although I refused to receive general anesthesia, I finally required sedation for the duration of the procedure because of my difficulty in breathing through the tracheotomy tube. I woke up shortly after the procedure and was happy to converse with the friendly recovery room staff. Leaving the hospital directly from the recovery room made the experience especially easier this time. When the bandages over the incision site in my neck were removed a week later I was happy to see that the skin tag that had reminded me of my ordeal was gone.

When I had a recurrence of diverticulitis (an inflammation of a pouch in the intestinal wall) nineteen months after the major operation, my gastroenterologist recommended the elective removal of the affected area in order to avoid further recurrences which carry a higher risk of complications. However, I persuaded him to consider only medical therapy and to delay the surgery, perhaps avoiding it completely. I explained to him that I was not emotionally able to deal with another surgery at that time. The prospect of being admitted to the hospital and becoming incapacitated again was unacceptable to me, especially after the elective procedure on my finger. I also felt that, in contrast to cancer, an infection was something I could deal with. Furthermore, I thought- *why undergo elective surgery before I know that I am cancer free?* If recurrence of cancer would occur sometime soon, ridding myself of the diverticula would be inconsequential for long term survival. If I have no recurrence of cancer in the next three to five years, I will reconsider the need for surgery.

Chapter 18. Trial and Errors

One of the most difficult issues I had to deal with during the nine months following my surgery related to my ability to speak. I was unable to speak as long as I had the tracheostomy tube. Fortunately I did not need the tube after a few weeks and only placed it in during the night to prevent shrinking of the stoma. After an additional six weeks, I gradually stopped that as well. Once the tube was out, I could speak using my voice prosthesis. I covered the tracheostomy opening in my neck with a special round housing, glued it tightly, and placed a replaceable air filter (called Heat and Moisture Exchanger or HME) in the hole at the center of the housing. The filter cleans the inhaled air and can also act as a valve that occludes air passage when pressed on. By pressing the filter cover using a finger, the exhaled air is forced into my esophagus through the prosthesis that connects the two passages. The vibrations produced by the exhaled air in the esophagus are converted to actual voice by the pronunciations made by the mouth.

The daily placement of these items is performed every morning and took up to twenty minutes in the beginning. The process is quite tedious. I have first to clean the skin around the stoma with water and soap to remove skin oil and then dry it, clean it with alcohol, place a skin protecting solution on the area, and if I want extra adherence capability spread special glue. Between each step of this regimen, I have to wait for several minutes to allow the applied materials to dry.

Removal of the housing before going to sleep was also cumbersome in the beginning. After the housing is taken off, the skin has to be cleansed by a special solvent called "Remove," which has then to be wiped off with alcohol. Then, the skin has to be cleaned with water and soap and dried. I learned the hard way that following all these steps meticulously is very crucial, because any deviation can weaken the adherence of the housing to the neck's skin which leads to the diversion of the exhaled air through the broken seal and render speech impossible. For example, not cleaning the removal solution with alcohol can interfere with the ability of the glue to achieve a good seal.

I struggled for several months to achieve a good seal around the stoma. The seal would only last a relatively short period of time, and I had to reseal the stoma several times a day. This was very frustrating because I could not speak consistently and could not predict when and if I would lose the ability to speak.

I looked to my local speech therapist at the Army Hospital for some instructions, but she only gave me samples of supplies from one of the two companies that produce stoma housings and instructed me how to order more. She briefly talked to me about placing the housing but never actually showed me how. The problem in sealing was finally solved for me when I returned to see the SLP in New York about two months later. She actually showed me how to place and remove the housing. I realized that I was missing an essential part in cleaning the skin – the cleansing of the "Remove" solution from my skin with alcohol. Apparently, the leftover removal solution weakens the new seal and leads to its failure. Once I reverted to wiping off the solution with alcohol and also washing the skin with soap prior to attaching the housing, it stayed on throughout the day and, on many occasions, even lasted longer. When my neck swelling subsided, I was able to achieve even better results.

I was amazed to find out how missing what seemed a simple technicality could lead to so much frustration and so many months of difficulties. When I mentioned this to my local SLP, she told me that she has never heard about this technique. It was one of the examples of how different SLPs are in their techniques and how this specialty is not only a science, but also an art. Another reason why my local SLP was unaware of this was because she was much less experienced than the one in New York. This experience underscores how post-operative care for tracheostomy patients needs to be better developed and standardized. A handbook or "best practices" guide is badly needed to inform all patients, surgeons, and SLPs about the simple steps that lead to a successful recovery.

Ordering the supplies I needed for maintaining my airways required contacting the supply companies on a regular basis. There were standard items that I needed, but also multiple types of housing items, and I was unsure which ones were the best for me. Medicare covered the basics supplies, but I had to pay the difference in price for items with better features. Because I experienced difficulties in sealing the housing, I tried several types at the suggestion of my local SLP. I finally found adequate items that helped me get a better seal with the help of the SLP from New York. After a few months I learned that as a veteran I am entitled to receive all my supplies from the local VA Hospital which made the process much easier.

About ten weeks after my surgery, my local SLP suggested I try to use a hands-free filter-valve system, which could enable me to speak without pushing down on the filter cover with my finger. This would free my hand and allow me to behave more naturally. I obtained a system and was elated to be able to feel the greater freedom it offered me. The disadvantage of the system was that it required more effort to speak and a stronger seal, and using it could break the housing seal. To prevent early breakage of the seal it has to be strongly glued to the neck's skin using special skin glue, which in turn takes more time and can also lead to irritation of the skin.

The other problem I had was with the actual plastic tracheo-esophageal voice prosthesis – a small tube that has a one-way valve at its esophageal end which allows air to enter the esophagus but prevents liquids or food from going the other direction into the trachea. If the valve does not close tightly, material can enter the trachea and the lungs. When that happens, fluids can spill through the prosthesis into the lungs, generating intense coughing while the body attempts to expel the aspirated material out of the lungs. The prosthesis is supposed to last for three to six months (and sometimes longer), but it failed in my case because of fluid leak after only seven to twenty-one days. What generally causes the valve to fail by not closing tightly is a piece of food or secretion or a buildup of yeast around the esophageal opening. The prosthesis can be flushed with water or brushed to try to clean it, but if this fails, it has to be replaced.

Unfortunately, most of my voice prosthesis failures happened over the weekends, and because the SLPs are not available during that time, I had to wait until Monday or even longer to have it changed. Replacing the voice prosthesis with a new one takes fifteen to thirty minutes and is an uncomfortable procedure. It involves pulling out the old prosthesis, inserting a plastic dilator into the hole in the trachea, leaving it there for about five minutes, and than reinserting a new one.

My first voice prosthesis failure occurred on a Friday evening only three weeks after its insertion. I noticed intense coughing when I drank and I observed in the mirror that drops of water were dripping down from the center of the prosthesis into my trachea. I almost panicked when it happened because I had no idea what I should do or how I could continue to eat or drink. I called my local surgeon at his home, and he told me to go to the emergency room where the on-call otolaryngology resident would remove the prosthesis and insert a small catheter in its hole to prevent it from sealing off until I could be seen by the SLP. Fortunately, I remembered that the SLP in New York had given me a special plug that could be placed in the voice prosthesis to temporarily stop the leakage. The trade-off was that I could no longer speak. I was able to locate the plug but found that it was slightly torn. I used superglue to seal the break in the plug and was able to stop the leakage until I got a new voice prosthesis on Monday.

As time passed and I had more leaks such as that one, I gradually learned not to panic but tried to cope with the leaks by consuming only semi-solid food or mixing any liquid with chewed food, making it less likely to drip into my lungs.

Both local and New York SLPs told me that it is common for voice prosthesis to fail immediately after the surgery. However, the problem did not resolve over time, and my surgeons were unable to advise me how to deal with it. My local surgeon had little experience and knowledge of how to effectively manage voice prosthesis problems and could not help me. I resorted to searching the medical literature in an effort to help myself. I quickly discovered that this topic is frequently discussed and that there are well tested methods to deal with it. Apparently, many otolaryngologists leave the care of this aspect of their patients to SLPs and are therefore inexperienced.

I shared the articles I found in the literature with him, the other local surgeon who had operated on me and my local SLP. While my surgeon welcomed the information I sent him he informed me that the other surgeon and my SLP did not welcome the information and were "insulted" by my attempt to "educate" them. I was stunned by this response. I had always believed in sharing information with my colleagues. Apparently these caregivers felt that my attempt to provide them with the most current literature was a sign of mistrust and not a genuine sharing of knowledge that could improve their abilities to provide better care.

My local SLP had no answer as to why my voice prosthesis kept failing and made no attempt to understand why they malfunctioned by examining them after she removed them unless I asked her to do so. I decided to find the cause of these failures myself, and when I looked at an extracted voice prosthesis under an operating microscope, I observed small particles of debris on its valve which prevented it from closing snugly. I swabbed that area and submitted it for culture to see if any organism could be identified. Even though the microbiology laboratory isolated yeast from the prosthesis, the SLP refused to recommend that I use antifungal agents and wanted me to wait and see if the next prosthesis would last longer. Unfortunately, it did not. She finally agreed that I should start using an antifungal agent after my SLP and surgeon in New York recommended it. Unfortunately, this did not help in prolonging the lifespan of the voice prosthesis.

In my desperation, I consulted with other SLPs over the internet or phone and posed inquiries on the internet site www.webwhispers. com, where laryngectomee patients share experiences and help each other. Although other individuals had a similar problem, no one had come up with a workable solution. When I saw the SLP in New York, she replaced my prosthesis with one that was resistant to colonization by yeast, but this one also failed after a few days. She tagged me as "a leaker," suggesting that I belong to an unlucky group of patients that have repeated failures of their voice prosthesis because of valve malfunction. Her attitude was that the solution to problems is through trial and error and that, eventually, a solution would be found. Her only suggestion was that I try to use a voice prosthesis made by another company or use a prosthesis that I could take out myself and clean. However, such prosthesis needed to be removed, cleaned, and reinserted at least once a week. I was not enthusiastic to revert to this type of prosthesis because it required wearing a safety attachment on the neck which can interfere with attaining a tight seal and because I did not want to repeatedly traumatize my stoma with weekly manipulations. It seemed that I was doomed to have a real problem in maintaining my ability to speak.

To my growing frustration, my local SLP did not respond to many of my email inquiries or phone calls. Finally, she sent me an email after I complained to the head of the department of otolaryngology. She demanded that I not contact her by email or phone but make an official appointment whenever I had a problem because she had a very busy schedule. This was so different from the attitude of my SLP in New York, who talked to me over the phone and promptly responded to my email inquiries. Her response aggravated my distress because I had no one to turn to locally. Her attitude was very different from any of the other SLPs I had encountered before or later, as all were very helpful and forthcoming and understood my emotional strain and the need for guidance and assistance.

The knowledge that help is readily available at all times is so essential for laryngectomees – especially new ones such as myself who experience difficulties after such a major life-changing experience.

After the SLP contacted my social worker and discussed this issue with her, she changed her attitude somewhat. I was happy to see her eventually leave the hospital. I was taken care from then onward by her replacement, who had an entirely different attitude that was similar to that of the SLP in New York. It was a welcome change and a great relief.

The repeated failures of my voice prosthesis made me fearful of traveling out of town because I was afraid that leakage might occur and that I would need the help of a SLP. When I traveled to Los Angeles to visit my daughter, who had just delivered a baby, I secured a SLP in the area and brought an extra voice prosthesis with me in case I needed replacement. When I planned a trip overseas, I contacted otolaryngologists in the countries I was to visit to ask their help in finding a local SLP in case I needed one.

To my pleasant surprise, I seemed to have alleviated my problem myself. My problem resolved unexpectedly because of an accidental discovery. During my stay in New York at my daughter's apartment, I used warm water to flush my prosthesis to relieve a sudden leakage. I had never used warm water before and always flushed the prosthesis twice a day as instructed by my SLPs with room-temperature tap water. To my relief, the leak ceased and did not come back. I decided to revert to using warm water to flush my prosthesis and had no leakages thereafter. My voice prosthesis last now much longer and often continues working for al least six months. I no longer use antifungal agents routinely because they did not prevent failures. However, I do use them whenever I take broad spectrum antibiotics because they promote colonization of the mouth with yeasts. I assume that the warm water is more effective in cleansing the prosthesis from food debris and dried mucus and may even impede the growth of yeast.

This simple solution altered my life. I feel a great sense of relief and freedom and no longer fear drinking because of a sudden need to cough after a sip of water. I still carry an extra prosthesis when I leave town but feel more secure in traveling. I was amazed that none of the SLPs with whom I consulted suggested this simple solution. In an attempt to help other patients, I informed my SLPs and surgeons about this method, as well the readers of the internet site for laryngectomees. I also posted my suggestions at a permanent internet site that advises laryngectomees and sent a brief explanation about it in the form of a "Letter to the Editor" to an otolaryngology journal. I was very pleased to see it published there so that surgeons and speech pathologists can use this simple method to help their patients. I am not sure if this method is the solution for all voice prosthesis leakages, but because it is so simple, I suggest that people try it. The only caution I added to my messages was to only use warm water and avoid hot water so as not to burn the esophagus. This can be done by first sipping the water. Several laryngectomees told me that they had also been using warm water with great success, and others told me that since they converted to using this method, they do not experience as many failures of their voice prosthesis.

Even though I have managed to figure out how to make my voice prosthesis last longer, failures still occur – sometimes at very inconvenient moments. On a trip to Los Angeles for my granddaughter's first birthday, my prosthesis started leaking just as I arrived for a one week stay. I called a local SLP whom I knew, but was told that she was away for four days. In my desperate attempt to find help, I called the local Veteran's Administration hospital where I had done my fellowship training some 35 years ago. I assumed that a medical center which serves many people with throat cancer would have an experienced SLP on staff. The hospital operator directed my call to the speech therapy department, but to my disappointment my phone call was answered by an answering machine and I was told to leave a message.

I was very frustrated, as it was Thursday afternoon and I knew I had to find help before the weekend or face continuous coughing and fluid aspiration. I remembered that I had the email address of another SLP in one of the medical centers in town. I sent her a message and was fortunate to get a call from her within thirty minutes. Yes, she could see me on Friday afternoon. My wife and I traveled across town to see her and she changed the voice prosthesis, thus reversing my agony and allowing me to eat and drink again without aspiration. Words can not express my gratitude to the SLP for her prompt assistance during a very busy working day. Her help and kind reassurance enabled me to continue my stay in Los Angeles and participate in the family celebration. Ironically, just as I returned from the SLP's office, I found a message from the SLP at the local Veterans Administration Hospital who also offered her assistance and even gave me her cell phone number so that I could call her after working hours. I was again moved by the kindness and helpfulness demonstrated by all of these professionals.

As had been the case after the removal of the initial cancer two years earlier, I was to be followed up once a month in the Otolaryngology Clinic to ensure that there was no recurrence. I was followed initially by one of the two surgeons who performed the three endoscopic surgeries in Washington. Even though I still felt disappointment and anger at their failure to remove the cancer initially, his dedication, emotional support, sincere care, and friendliness helped me overcome the difficulties and problems I encountered. His door was always open to me, and he acted immediately to assist me in any way he could. I walked into his office several times a week – sometimes just to speak with him and tell him how I was doing. He hugged me every time I left, which made me feel that I had a true friend that cared for me. On several occasions, he reacted to my complaints with exaggerated vigor and often performed tests that could have been delayed. In retrospect, he might have felt over-vigilant because of the friendship we developed. I was very sad to see him leave when he was called to serve in Afghanistan for eight months. After his departure, I was followed for several months by the other surgeon who had operated on me, but he, too, was sent on a duty tour, this time to Iraq.

I saw Dr. Marker in New York several times after my surgery. I asked him to recommend a civilian otolaryngologist in Washington for me to see so that I did not have to travel to New York as often. I realized that I could not have continuity of care in a military facility, especially during war time, and I wanted to be seen by someone with greater experience in my type of cancer. Since the local otolaryngologists had only limited experience in managing patients with my type of cancer I felt the need to be followed by a more seasoned one.

He recommended such an expert, and I saw him every few months for follow-up thereafter. This enabled me to travel to New York City for medical care less often.

The importance of experience in follow-up was vividly illustrated on several occasions. When my first MRI and CT scans after the surgery were performed, the radiologists and otolaryngologists at the military hospitals were concerned about some abnormalities they observed in the scans. I sent these scans to Dr. Marker, and he assured me that such findings are common after extensive surgery and that they did not signify a return of the malignancy. His interpretation was based on many such surgeries and withstood the test of time.

Another issue where experience truly counted was the assessment of my swallow test. Because I was still experiencing difficulty in swallowing food two months after my surgery, my local otolaryngologist ordered a swallow test. The test encompasses ingesting radio-opaque material, and the passage of the material is monitored using X-rays. The SLP who performed the test, as well as the otolaryngologist, interpreted the test results as showing that I had significant narrowing in the esophagus that required mechanical dilatation. Such narrowing is common after the kind of surgery I had, due to scarring. The dilation is a procedure where a series of tubes with larger diameters are inserted into the esophagus, often under anesthesia, which breaks down the scarring. However, it often causes pain and in many cases needs to be repeated because the narrowing recurs.

At my request, my otolaryngologist called Dr. Marker and asked his advice as to whether or not dilatation is permissible so soon after surgery. Dr. Marker, who could not review the actual study and relied on the information he received by phone, assured my surgeon, "If significant narrowing is present, this procedure is permissible." Fortunately, the other local surgeon recommended waiting another month before performing the dilatation. I saw Dr. Marker three weeks later and showed him the video of the swallow test. He, as well as his SLP, conclusively excluded any significant esophageal narrowing and assured me that the stricture I had was expected at this time after the surgery and would improve over time. They also observed that much of the swallowing difficulty was caused by a longer-than-necessary prosthesis that was protruding into the esophagus and blocking the passage of food. After the SLP replaced the voice prosthesis with a shorter one, my swallowing improved. Dr. Marker was also correct that the swallowing would improve over time. I felt fortunate that I saw Dr. Marker before the scheduled dilatation and was subsequently able to avoid it.

This incident, as well others, illustrated to me the importance of continuity of care by experienced clinicians after major surgery such as I had. While Dr. Marker, an expert who specializes in the field, was very familiar with the long-term follow-up and the potential long-term problems, the less experienced local surgeons were less able to deal with these.

Chapter 19. Is it Cancer Again?

Life after the removal of my larynx was different. I had to deal with new practical problems like re-learning how to eat and speak, but I also confronted a difficult emotional obstacle: the constant fear that the cancer may return. I will discuss the eating and speaking issues in the following chapters, but first I want to address my anxiety about the cancer's return.

The fear that I was not cured was hanging over me at all times. I was afraid to make long-term plans such as taking an out of town trip to visit my children. When confronted with a simple task like sorting my mail, I tried to finish it promptly in case I got sick again. Once a month, I visited the Otolaryngology Clinic for an examination of my throat and had PET-CT scans every three months for the first year and less often later. Each night before the scans, I became nervous. I remembered what it was like when I had my second scan three years before and the anxiety it produced because of the suspicious findings. After the scan was complete, I would linger in the hospital, eagerly awaiting the results. On several occasions, these tests showed worrisome findings that necessitated further studies; and in other instances, they manifested inconclusive results that had to be monitored until the next scans, planting a seed of uncertainty in my mind. Whenever the scans did not show any new abnormality, I felt great relief and that I had been granted a temporary lease on life until the next tests were done. My life became a series of three-month intervals of relative calm until the next set of scans.

I was eventually told by my otolaryngologist sixteen months after my last surgery that there was no need to repeat the scans so often because they were stable and did not show any ominous signs of cancerous spread. He recommended that these scans would be done at six to twelve months intervals because there is no scientific evidence that repeating them at three month interval improve survival and it is just a waste of medical resources. What he was also attempting to tell me without actually saying it was that if the cancer did spread to other locations in my body, there was little that could be done to combat it, and knowing about it earlier would not change the outcome. He explained, "You had extensive surgery that removed all the cancer, and there is very good chance that you are actually cured. However, remember that spread and recurrences can still occur, especially in the first five years, and therefore you need to be physically examined every six to eight weeks."

I was hesitant to accept this message. I became so used to the three-month cycle of scans, which was actually recommended by my physicians because of suspicious findings that eventually disappeared. I had to accept the reality that I would always have to live with the threat of cancer's return and that physical examination and vigilance would be the best ways of monitoring my condition. Accepting this was difficult, but eventually it partially freed me from the endless cycle of scans that was accompanied by anxiety prior to the tests and temporary relief after they came back negative.

Following the major surgery, I experienced constant and non-relenting medical problems that plagued me. I was afraid of the worst-case scenario. For each ailment, regardless of its severity, my mind jumped to the conclusion that the problems were the result of the cancer spreading locally or systemically. This snowballing of anxiety and worry was only relieved after I underwent thorough medical evaluation, including radiological and other studies. After so many close calls, I refused to let my guard down and believe again that the cancer was gone.

The first of these ailments that sparked my concern was the reemergence of migraine headaches that had disappeared after my laryngectomy surgery. I had no explanation for the disappearance of the migraines but was happy to enjoy the respite I got after a lifelong affliction with them. I joked about God having pity on me and freeing me from headaches because I had endured so many different kinds of pain and discomfort. A potential reason for the disappearance of headaches was that I could no longer breathe through my nose and therefore was not able to smell odors that triggered my migraines.

I was happy to regain some ability to smell about three months after the surgery. Unfortunately, with the renewed smelling capacity my susceptibility to migraines returned. However, I did not make this association right away, and when the first headache did not abate after eight days, I was very concerned and worried that it was due to a serious problem, such as the spread of the cancer to the brain, even though my surgeons assured me that my type of cancer rarely disseminates there. I tried to see a neurologist but could not get an appointment right away and was sent to the Emergency Room. The doctor there did not suspect such a complication, but because she understood my anxieties, she ordered a head CT right away and an MRI scan, which was performed a few days later. Happily, both were normal.

My internist diagnosed mild anemia a short time after my last surgery. Even though this was likely related to the blood loss I incurred during the surgeries, the multiple blood drawings I had, and my deficient diet, I was worried that it was due to the persistence of the malignancy or an intestinal bleed. I also had an unexplained blood test finding of an elevated sedimentation rate, which is a nonspecific sign of abnormality. My doctor suggested that we wait and see if these issues would resolve by themselves, but sensing my anxiety, she ordered abdominal MRI and CT scans, which did not show any sign of malignancy. Both of these issues resolved on their own within a few months.

About the same time, on a Saturday morning, I noticed the appearance of a new skin rash on my thighs. I became very distressed and knew I had to wait until Monday to see a dermatologist. I was fortunate that a dermatologist I knew had a clinic on Saturdays.

He was gracious and agreed to see me, even though he had a full clinic. After examining me, he performed a biopsy of the skin and assured me that the rash was not of a serious nature. The biopsy confirmed his initial assessment; however, in about ten percent of patients, this kind of rash is known to be associated with the presence of a malignancy somewhere in the patient. This was troubling news. Again, there was uncertainty whether I was actually cured. I had to get used to this reality, but my dermatologist reminded me that in ninety percent of the patients, the cause of this rash remains unknown. I was hoping to be one of those. This rash recurred for several months, reigniting my worry every time it reappeared. About ten months later, it finally disappeared.

To compound this, a new type of rash appeared two weeks later. This time, I went to the Dermatology Clinic in the hospital, and the biopsy they took showed a rare type of rash that was suggestive of leukemia of the skin. However, the dermatologist was not completely sure and wanted to wait a month and repeat the biopsy. A month of worry passed by before a repeat biopsy showed that the lesion was benign. I was relieved but realized that my anxieties were not over yet, and any new medical issue would generate suspicion and worry.

My earlier experiences with the pathological results of biopsies made me very sensitive to their interpretation. When, at my urging, my dermatologist performed a biopsy of a suspicious skin lesion and promised to call me about the results in five to six days, I was not particularly concerned until I heard the message his secretary left on my answering machine. Instead of telling me the results or reassuring me that "everything is fine," she asked me to call back. My previous experience with an otolaryngologist who did not tell me the ominous results over the phone made me very concerned. I was afraid that I would again hear bad news. What made this especially stressful was that I received the call on Yom Kippur, the holiest day in the Jewish calendar, while in the synagogue. I immediately called my dermatologist but unfortunately he could not talk to me right away as he was busy performing procedures. Since I wanted to return to the services in the synagogue, I parked myself at a location in the prayer hall close to the exit where there was good phone reception. I placed my phone on a vibration mode and waited.

While waiting for the call I thought that it was so ironic that, on a day where Jews believe that God decides who is going to live and who is going to die, I was anticipating a notification of my own fate. When my dermatologist finally called and said that the lesion was only premalignant, I was relieved. Yes, it was not a benign finding and the lesion needed to be observed for a while, but it was not cancer. Being vigilant worked again.

About ten months after my last surgery, I started to experience pain on the left side of my jaw. I first suspected it to be caused by a problem with my temporal mandibular joint, but my dentist did not confirm it and just adjusted my bite. Because the pain did not abate, I sought the help of my otolaryngologists, who did not find anything that could explain the pain. Since all my PET scans performed after my surgeries showed increased metabolic activity in the left side of my head, they were concerned that the pain was related to something serious and ordered new CT and MRI scans.

The MRI showed a suspicious area at the base of the skull, but that was inconclusive. However, there were no signs of cancer-like lesions at that area, and they decided to repeat the MRI after a month. The otolaryngologists explained that the suspected area is very difficult to biopsy because it is located at the base of the skull; therefore, it is best to wait and observe. Besides, they elaborated, if indeed my cancer had spread to other areas, any invasive procedure that carried high morbidity was not worth pursuing because surgical access to that area was very difficult. I realized that each diagnostic test and procedure might be the start of a long road toward more cancer treatments – or worse.

At about the time the jaw pain appeared, I was planning to leave on my first overseas trip since the surgeries. Prior to the cancer ordeal, I had traveled all over the world frequently, not giving much thought to taking a flight to China or India. Now that I was scheduled to deliver lectures in Turkey and Israel, I considered canceling. Even without the challenges of delivering a lecture with my new voice, I was concerned about the enduring complications from my surgeries.

I hesitated to take the trip, fearing that my medical problems would only worsen. However, since I secured medical care of experienced specialists and speech pathologists in both countries, I decided to take the chance and travel. Throughout my career, I have taken pride in honoring my commitments to deliver lectures despite occasional scheduling conflicts, medical problems, or personal inconveniences. I did not want to start a new trend of becoming a "no show" at the conferences and institutes which had invited me.

To my great surprise, I tolerated the six flights and airport changes and very much enjoyed my trip. My presentations on both trips were successful, and I spent a few days in Turkey and was able to enjoy touring several archeological sites in the vicinity of the town where I stayed and enjoyed the hospitality of my hosts.

The trip to Israel was most enjoyable, and I visited many friends and family I had not seen for over three years. For most of my relatives and friends there, it was the first time they had seen me after my surgeries. Some confided with me about serious medical problems they had for a while. Apparently, they had felt that by sharing these with me, they could show how they overcame and learned to accept them. I was welcomed with love and appreciation for the efforts I made to travel and even found time to sightsee and visit places I had not been before.

My facial pain continued throughout the trip, and I was unsure whether I should seek medical care in Israel. Since my time there was short and my agenda so full, I kept postponing it, even though some of my physician friends offered to examine and treat me if needed. About a week into my trip, I noticed that the diffuse pain had become concentrated at one location near the upper molar tooth on the left side. For years, I'd had various dental issues, but for the first time, I was happy to have one because the alternative was cancer. I was glad that I had listened to my otolaryngologists and did not exert pressure on them to perform invasive procedures to get to the bottom of the problem. What happened illustrates that time is often the best medicine. I suspected that I had a cracked tooth and started myself on antibiotics to reduce the intensity of the infection and perhaps control the pain. I wondered if some of the increased uptake observed by the recent PET scans might have been caused by an infection associated with the fractured tooth. To my relief, the pain subsided within thirty-six hours and became tolerable. The response to the antibiotics strengthened my assertion that this was, indeed, a dental infection and nothing more.

Upon my return to Washington, I immediately sought the help of a dentist, who confirmed that the painful tooth was indeed cracked. After several attempts to treat that tooth failed, it was pulled out, and the pain slowly subsided and disappeared. Although the recovery and healing took almost three weeks (which was longer than I experienced after I had other teeth pulled out prior to receiving radiation), I was happy to put this anxiety-causing problem behind me. The changes in the PET scans that had caused so much anxiety also disappeared three months later, confirming their connection to the dental problem.

The new symptoms that kept emerging took an emotional toll on me. I was frustrated and tired of the endless cycle of new problems that did not abate. It seemed that I had no respite from medical problems. Once one of them resolved, a new one would emerge. I was yearning for normality and peace of mind but could not get it. Monitoring myself so closely and getting to the bottom of each problem became a full-time job for me.

My worries about cancer in the oral cavity rose again three months later when during a routine dental cleaning, the dental hygienist noticed a small hole-like lesion on my gums above a dental implant. Even though the dentist who looked at it assured me that this was most probably due to local infection or trauma, my first question to him was if it could be due to a cancerous lesion. I openly admitted to him that I was fearful of cancer and had exaggerated anxiety about it.

I had a respite from medical problems for a week before another one emerged. This time, it was pain in my left chest, sometimes very intense. I was worried that the pain might be caused by a lesion that was cancerous or cardiac in nature. There were many signs, however, that the pain was muscle related and not cardiac in origin. This was because the chest muscles and ribs were sensitive to pressure, and the pain was exacerbated when I used my chest muscles, especially when I was breathing deeply. However, I was not entirely sure.

I chose to keep the existence of the pain to myself and not share it with my wife because I wanted to spare her the worry. I did not want her to go through another pain saga with me. When I sought medical attention, the internist excluded heart problems and agreed with me that the pain was probably muscular in nature.

I suspected that the pain was a side effect of a medication that lowers cholesterol levels (a statin) that I had begun taking about ten days prior to the beginning of the pain. Muscle pain is the major side effect of this class of agents. When I stopped taking the statin, the pain disappeared within forty-eight hours, thereby confirming my suspicion.

Again, I was free of medical worries for only a short time until the time came to repeat my routine PET and MRI scans. The PET scan did not show any new findings, and even the previously observed enhanced uptake was reduced in intensity, although not entirely gone. The MRI was performed on Saturday, and early Monday morning, I went to the Neuro-Radiology office to talk to the radiologists about their interpretations of the scan. The head of the department was always very helpful and accommodating in reviewing the scans with me. He had already reviewed the scans and informed me that he did not see any mass at the area of the metabolic enhanced area detected by the PET scan. This was very good news. However, there was a new and concerning finding – a lesion on the left collar bone (clavicle) that had not been seen before. He asserted that since there was no enhanced metabolic activity detected at that location in the PET scan, the new lesion might be a nonmalignant or a nonaggressive tumor. He called the expert who read the PET scan to confirm this. Even though this was not a typical site for neck cancer metastasis, which usually appears in the lungs and liver, he recommended that the lesion should be biopsied.

Even though the information I received was not too ominous, I was shaken by this news. *Does it mean that the cancer has spread? Is everything I went through until now in vain? Is all the progress that I've made going to matter now? Why take statin now to prevent heart disease if the cancer has spread? Why worry about replacing the tooth that I just lost? Will I live long enough to finish writing this book? I probably will not be able to travel and see my new granddaughter and family as I had planned.*

Suddenly, all my priorities changed, and I was facing my worst nightmare... *The Genie is out of the box because the cancer has spread to the bone.* I wanted to find out what was going on as soon as possible. I knew, however, that it might be some time before I could get a definite answer.

I did not show any outward signs of distress, even though I felt very worried and concerned. I asked the radiologist if this lesion should be biopsied right away. He agreed and suggested I get my otolaryngologist to order a biopsy, after which he would help me have it done as soon as possible. He assured me again that even if it was cancer, the likelihood that it was a very aggressive one was low.

I immediately went over to the Otolaryngology Clinic to ask my doctors to order a biopsy. Unfortunately, they were in the operating room and were not due to return until the afternoon. I felt the urgency to get the biopsy done as soon as possible and did not want to wait until they finished the surgeries. I approached another staff member who was in the clinic that day, and he was very kind and helpful in reading the MRI himself and agreed that a biopsy should be done. When he proceeded to order the biopsy, I asked him to make the order urgent. He complied and proceeded to calm my anxiety by explaining to me that such a bone lesion might be caused by the radiation I had previously received and might not be cancerous at all. This was very reassuring and comforting, and I hoped that he would be proven correct.

When I returned to the neuro-radiologist's office and informed him that the biopsy was ordered, he contacted the interventional radiologist, who promised to review my MRI and call me to schedule a CT-guided biopsy. He was hoping to do it even on that day, but definitely within a week.

I did not wait but went up to the interventional radiologist's office, where I introduced myself and briefly described to him my medical history and previous illness. He appreciated my distress at the uncertainty of the finding and offered to perform the biopsy as soon as possible. Fortunately, the CT equipment was available within one and a half hours. He inquired if I had recently eaten, in case I would need systemic intravenous sedating medications. I reassured him that I would not require any of these medications and that I could cope with the procedure without them. His assessment of the low density of the lesion was that it was not made of bone but was fatty in nature, which was reassuring.

At the CT facility I had to lay flat without any movement for the entire thirty minutes that it took to complete the biopsy. I was fortunate not to have eaten or drunk anything for about five hours, because there were no stomach contents that could regurgitate to my mouth. However, it was hard for me to lie flat because my oral secretions accumulated in my mouth and mucus collected at my trachea. I was trying very hard not to cough throughout the procedure.

Fortunately, the involved bone was close to the skin and could be easily reached by using a short biopsy needle. I was apprehensive lying down and waiting for the painful procedure. I was worried about being stuck by a large needle that would be inserted into my chest. I also wondered whether I should have asked for sedation that would calm me down or even help me forget this experience. I decided to tough it out and showed no signs of distress. I knew that the accuracy of the procedure depended, to a large extent, on my calmness and cooperation. I wanted to experience the procedure, be alert enough to understand it, ask questions, deal with the results, and assure that the specimens were read and diagnosed with as little delay as possible.

It was after numbing the skin and the outer layer of the bone that the doctor inserted the biopsy needle and pierced the bone. I felt little pain throughout the procedure. He performed several CT scans to assure that the needle was inserted into the affected area in the bone.

The aspirated material was liquid, bloody, and had no hard tumor-like consistency. This was very reassuring. I studied the aspirated material under the microscope with the doctor and saw only blood cells and no others cells that could represent cancer. Of course, this was not a definite diagnosis but was a good finding. The specimens were sent to the pathology laboratory to be stained and studied.

I was so relieved to learn that the biopsy most likely revealed no cancer and glad to be free of all the doomsday worries and potential catastrophe. I was almost euphoric with joy. I suddenly had a new lease on life. I expressed my deep appreciation to the interventional radiologist and told him how helpful he was in finding out the true nature of the lesion and sparing me the anxiety and fear I would have to endure should I have had to wait a longer time. It was amazing, I told him that three and a half hours after learning about the suspicion of cancer, a biopsy was performed and read, and my fear of doomsday was gone. He responded, "This is the way it should be in any good medical center." He also told me that he very much appreciated my gratitude, which made his work worthwhile.

After I learned about the good news, I personally informed the otolaryngologist and neuro-radiologist about them and thanked them for their help. I talked briefly with my radiation oncologist, who explained to me that a cystic-like degenerative lesion as I had can indeed occur in irradiated bones. My last stop was in the pathology laboratory, where I found the pathologist who was to read my biopsy. I told him jokingly, "I have had bad news on my past two visits to the pathology laboratory and hope for good news this time." "However," I told him "I want to know the truth whatever it is," He promised to call me on the next day with the results.

Even though I believed that the pathological results would show no cancer, I was not completely sure and waited anxiously for the call from the pathologist. The confirmatory phone call came twenty-four hours later. The pathologist reported that the aspirated material contained only blood, and there was no cancer to be found.

The day of learning about the potential spread of the cancer followed by the final relief was very draining and exhausting. I shared that morning's experiences with my wife only when she came back from work. I was happy to have been able to handle it myself and spare her the tension and uncertainty. I elected to spare my children from these events, at least for the present time.

When I shared the day's events with my otolaryngologist, he told me that my experience is common to many other patients with cancer who keep living through these stressful events for the rest of their lives. They suspect cancer to be the culprit of every new physical, radiological, or laboratory finding. "You will have to learn to live and better cope with this reality." he concluded. I hoped to live long enough to experience this. I also felt very tired of these unrelenting medical and dental problems and hoped to finally have a peaceful period.

Over time, I have begun to get used to these unexpected stressful events, even though they take their toll on me. My knowledge in medicine makes me more aware of the potential significance of new and alarming findings. However, I realized that I tend to catastrophize them and generally assume the worse. Over time, I became more rational in my approach and generally wait and think about the situation and new findings more carefully before rushing to fully investigate them by going to experts and consultants and getting new blood tests and scans. I am, however, still vigilant and am driven by the quest to stay healthy and alive by trying to fix and get to the bottom of any new medical problem.

Chapter 20. Eating

Eating became a major stumbling block after my laryngectomy. I lost about ten pounds over the months of the radiation treatment and surgeries and slowly regained that weight after I recovered. In retrospect, having some weight to lose was an asset, because it allowed me to draw energy and nutrients from my body stores. It was almost like using your life savings during difficult financial times. I was always concerned about becoming overweight, but realized now that in my state of health, having some extra weight could prove helpful.

I did not appreciate how I missed eating until I could not eat anything by mouth after my major surgery. During that time, I frequently had dreams about eating and worried that I had harmed myself. I gradually regained my ability to eat again through a slow and tedious process that took several months. It took a long time because the swelling in my newly formed esophagus had to decrease so that food could pass through. Initially, I was allowed and only able to ingest liquids, but I slowly progressed to semi-solid and finally more solid food.

As time passed, I was slowly able to eat almost any food as long as I chewed it thoroughly and mixed it with liquid in my mouth prior to swallowing. The water or other drinks decreased the viscosity of the food. Liquids enhanced the swallowing because the transplanted flap that formed my new larynx lacked peristaltic activity, and therefore could not propel the food downward towards my stomach. I am still unable to ingest unpeeled apples or large pills because they get stuck in my throat. It is also difficult and time consuming for me to eat hard food such as meat and I avoid it if possible. Finding the right dish in a restaurant is challenging because I try to avoid spicy or dry food items. I have to chew large pills or pour the contents of capsules to a spoon so that I can swallow them. Trying to eat vegetables or oranges is challenging but eventually achievable.

Because I have to consume a lot of fluids with my food, I quickly get filled up and can only eat small amounts of food each time. Since water gets absorbed from the stomach rather rapidly, I end up feeling hungry every two hours. Drinking so much liquid is cumbersome at times, and I need many water refills when I eat in restaurants. The excess fluid ingestions send me to the bathroom frequently during the day and night. Since my surgery, I visit the bathroom about every two hours during the night and often wake up in the morning rather sleep deprived.

The process of eating takes a long time. I changed from the one who finishes his food first to the one who finishes last. Now, everyone waits for me to end my meal. My ingestion is gravity dependent and food would come back into my mouth if I leaned forward. I learned that I could not bend forward after eating or drinking, or what I ate would come back into my mouth.

One of the changes that occurred after my radiation and surgeries was the diminishment of my ability to smell and taste. I could not smell at all after the surgery because I no longer moved air through my nose. I was not aware of this initially but had a wide awakening when the fire alarm in the house sounded several times because of burned toast. I was afraid that I could not smell a gas leak or early fire, and I often asked my wife to smell for me when I suspected a problem. There was one benefit of not being able to smell, and that was my complete freedom from chronic migraine headaches that were induced by fumes. Happily, though, I regained some ability to smell after a few months as I learned to assist myself in introducing air into my nose by closing my mouth and swallowing. However, with this regained sense, the migraines came back.

My taste that was lost almost completely after radiation returned slowly but was altered. The most annoying part was that the sensation to spices became magnified to the degree that even mildly spicy food became too hot. I often cannot eat food that tastes mild to others. This makes it difficult sometimes to choose food in a restaurants and hard for my wife to prepare food for me.

I learned that I cannot speak while swallowing because the food I swallow takes much longer to go down to my stomach. When I attempt to speak prematurely, my voice becomes muffled, and this sometimes causes leakage of fluid through my voice prosthesis into my trachea. This happens because food or fluid accumulates in my esophagus because of a narrowing near the TEP site. I actually feel air bubbling through the accumulated food. I have to apologize to those who eat with me that I cannot talk to them while I eat. I often cannot answer the phone because I am in the middle of eating and, even after I swallow the food, it takes me up to ten seconds before I can talk. I sometimes spit out the food from my mouth so that I can answer the phone.

I realized after a few months that my renewed ability to eat was fragile. I experienced a sudden inability to swallow in a most unfortunate time while on a trip to California about a year after my surgery. My wife and I were staying at a bed-and-breakfast in a small town in the mountains of San Andrea near Santa Barbara. While eating breakfast, I unexpectedly experienced great difficulty swallowing any solid food. The food eventually became stuck in my throat, and I was unable to swallow it or spit it out – similarly to what had happened in the first months after my laryngectomy. I hoped that I could relieve the obstruction by vomiting so that the stomach contents would push the stuck food from below. When I tried to explain to my wife what had happened, I discovered that I had no voice, probably because the stuck food was obstructing the air passages. I hand signaled to her that I was going to leave the dining room and return to our room and, fortunately, she understood.

After I got to the room, I attempted first to rinse my mouth and flush the voice prosthesis with warm water, but this did not help. Happily, I was able to relieve the obstruction by vomiting, but I found out when I tried to eat again that any food I ingested got stuck.

Fortunately, I was able to drink fluids again, although even this was uncomfortable. I was relieved, however, that at least I was able to keep myself hydrated. When I looked into my mouth through a mirror, I did not see anything abnormal. However, I could not look beyond the mouth.

I felt very upset as well as frightened at what had happened. I was in a predicament. We were in a remote mountain location with limited medical access. I had no idea what could be the cause of the sudden obstruction. I was trying to sort out the causes and wondered if this was caused by food stuck on the inner side of my prosthesis lodged in my esophagus and tried to rotate the voice prosthesis without any relief. I wondered if this is due to tissue swelling caused by food that was rough and induced local trauma, or perhaps because of local infection. However, I had no pain or sign of infection. It was reassured knowing that I was thoroughly examined by my otolaryngologist a week earlier. It was also comforting that my airways were permanently separated now from my esophagus, and there was no danger that I would suffocate.

Fortunately, this was early in the day on the East Coast, and I was able to reach my otolaryngologist in his office by phone. He suggested that I consume only liquids for the next day so that my upper digestive tract could rest from any possible trauma and that if I felt that I had anymore trouble, I should go to an emergency room. He assured me that he or one of his associates would see me in the clinic upon my return home, which was in three days. I was calmed and assured by his response and also knew that if I needed it, medical care was only about an hour away.

I restricted myself to fluids during the rest of the trip and did not alter our plans, which included hiking and biking. I consumed only liquid food such as buttermilk and soft drinks. I lost two pounds during those three days. On our flight back to Washington, I tried to eat a slice of bread since I could not bring any liquids to the plane. It was very difficult to swallow, even though I drank water with the bread. It took me about an hour to eat the bread.

Before going to the Otolaryngology Clinic, I attempted to eat some bread so that I could update my doctors about my situation. I was happy to note that swallowing felt easier. My surgeon was not there that morning, and a resident and a senior surgeon examined me. Their thorough examination (which included endoscopy) revealed no abnormality. Nevertheless, they immediately scheduled a radiological swallow test and a barium swallow study of my upper gastrointestinal tract. The swallow test revealed narrowing of my esophagus near the TEP site, but that had been observed before. Happily, the difficulty in swallowing that came so abruptly and lasted for four days subsided within a day, and no one was able to explain its origin. However, this incident served as a vivid reminder that my ability to swallow is not entirely assured.

Another incident that underscored my vulnerability occurred a few months later. My wife and I were traveling in Ireland and were having dinner in a restaurant in a remote, small seaside town. I was eating fish and was very careful to avoid any bones. While enjoying the good food, I suddenly felt pain in my throat. I must have missed a small fish bone that got stuck in my throat. I felt very helpless when it happened and did my best not to panic. I tried first to flush the bone by drinking water and eating bread and, when this did not work, I attempted in vain to see my throat in a mirror and remove the bone with a small forceps that I carry. Attempting to push food from my stomach to dislodge the bone did not work either.

I realized then that my "new throat," which is constructed of my forearm skin and therefore has no peristalsis that propels food down into the stomach, is very vulnerable to accidents such as the one I experienced. My wife suggested that I go to the closest emergency room. However, the restaurant owner informed us that this town had only a small hospital which was not staffed at night by doctors. The doctors would need to be contacted first before going to the hospital. Furthermore, there was no otolarygologist in the small town, and the only physicians there were general practitioners. The closest large medical center was three hours away and could only be reached through small rural roads. In preparation for our trip, I had contacted the head of the Department of Otolaryngology in Dublin should I have any problems, but this was five hours away.

I was fortunate that with the encouragement of the restaurant owner, I was finally able to remove the bone. I did it by eating dry bread without drinking water, which was very uncomfortable but probably generated the necessary friction to finally move the bone. Even though the painful sensation was finally gone, I was unsure if my efforts were successful because I still had discomfort in my throat. To our great relief, this also resolved in a day. After this incident, I avoided eating any fish and just consumed soft food or soups. I was not going to take any risks.

These experiences underscored how vulnerable I became and that I must now cope with the unknown elements of my new breathing and eating system. Venturing out in the world requires a leap of faith that things will work and that no unfortunate events will happen.

Chapter 21. Getting Emergency Care

I realized that, because I am a neck breather, I am at a high risk of receiving inadequate therapy when seeking urgent medical care. About nineteen months after my laryngectomy I experienced a sudden onset of shortness of breath. It was very frightening because I had never experience this before – and I was home alone when it happened. Rather than risk the delays potentially inherent in calling 911, I decided to drive to the closest community hospital, which was about two miles away. I felt that I needed to act quickly before my condition deteriorated.

When I arrived at the emergency room I attempted to explain the seriousness of my condition to the receptionist, but this was very difficult for me because of my shortness of breath. Fortunately, she seemed to understand and admitted me without any delay. When two nurses came into my room, I pointed to my stoma site and told them that it was difficult for me to breathe. This would not have been difficult to observe because I was breathing very fast, each breath labored and shallow.

I kept pointing to my tracheostomy site, hoping they would understand that I needed to get oxygen delivered in that location. The nurses finally understood that I needed oxygen only after I was able to utter a few words; they proceeded to place oxygen tubes into my nose, not realizing that I do not breathe through my nose but through my tracheostomy. It was very difficult for me to talk at that moment because I had to remove my HME filter so that I could inhale enough air. I kept placing the HME into my stoma so that I could speak a few words. It took about three minutes – which to me seemed like forever – until they understood my explanation and another three minutes for them to find an oxygen mask in the right size and deliver oxygen in the correct way. I was fortunate that the oxygen did help within a few minutes.

I was also having great difficulty in conveying my medical condition and relaying the list of medications I was receiving because I could not speak while receiving oxygen. I was finally able to supply this information in writing. I realized then that I should have such a list with me at all times. Not having it places me at great risk because it deprives any future caregiver of essential information.

It was a very scary and frustrating experience. I was at the very place where I should have been helped, yet the people who were entrusted with that task were unable to deliver it appropriately. I was fortunate that I was conscious and able to speak, but dread the thought of what would have happened if I were unable to communicate my needs. I realized that many emergency room personnel (and perhaps other first responders) do not recognize a patient who has had a laryngectomy and is a neck breather. This can lead to devastating consequences.

When I described what had happened to my otolaryngologist (who works at another hospital) this was his illuminating response:

"I am sorry you had a difficult experience. It is a terrible feeling to be in distress and not be able to communicate the correct action to people. With the significant success of laryngeal conservation treatment, we have fewer and fewer laryngectomy patients and it is becoming a rare medical condition. You might consider keeping a short document with you (like a bracelet) that explains your airway management."

I followed his advice and since that incident I wear a bracelet that states that I am a neck breather and a short written explanation regarding how oxygen should be delivered to me.

I also communicated my experience to the head of the Department of Otolaryngology at the hospital where I teach who responded.

"We hope that all MDs know how to recognize a laryngectomee. This, however, does not always happen. We try to educate where we can. I don't know if there is anything formal in the emergency room curriculum. I will forward you message to one of our lead emergency room doctors . . . ."

This experience brought home to me the need to do something to improve the education of health care providers so that they can avoid such mistakes and the resultant delays in appropriate care. It drove me to try to educate the emergency room personal in my area so that no other laryngectomees will endure what I had gone through.

The first hospital I contacted was the place where I originally sought care. Of course I had a personal motive - - knowing that this is the hospital to which I would probably turn should I need urgent medical care – but also to make sure the personnel there can help other laryngectomees. When I received no response from them after a week, I went there myself and asked to speak with the medical director of the emergency room. The director was very receptive to hearing what had happened to me and promised to convey it to the head nurse who supervises staff training. He assured me that this will be a topic in which they will all be retrained. I also personally visited both my local fire and police stations to inform them about my medical status.

I shared my experience with all the heads of the departments of otolaryngology and emergency rooms in my area. I offered to come in and personally demonstrate to the emergency room personnel how a laryngectomee looks and the proper way to resuscitate and deliver oxygen to them.

I also wrote a short essay for the International Association of Laryngectomees' Newsletter which described my experience and what others who are similarly situated can do to avoid it. I suggested not only that they wear a bracelet identifying them as neck breathers, but that they should also communicate their needs ahead of time by calling their local police and fire departments, as well as any supplemental local Emergency Response Teams. Patients, or their doctors, should contact the emergency rooms in their areas so that their personnel will be able to recognize and deliver assistance to a neck breather. They should also carry a short list describing their medical conditions, their medications, and the names of their doctors and contact information.

I realized that it up to us, as laryngectomees, to be vigilant and increase the awareness of medical personnel with whom we are likely to come into contact. Health care professionals vary in their degree of knowledge about our condition – and, of course, personnel change over time. Even though the care of neck breathers is taught at Cardio-Pulmonary Resuscitation courses, many caregivers are not familiar with this category of patients.

Chapter 22. How Others Treat Me

Looking and speaking differently from other people make me stand out. However, I elected not to hide the site of the filter (HME) that covers my stoma. The bottle cap sized plastic circle stands out quite prominently, right in the middle of my neck. Initially, I thought that I might wish to hide the HME by covering it with a scarf or other garment, but I realized soon that I could not do so because I need to have easy access to quickly remove it whenever I need to cough or sneeze. If I do not remove the HME promptly before I cough or sneeze, the filter becomes clogged with mucus and has to be replaced.

I was surprised that I am actually not ashamed or embarrassed wearing the HME filter on my neck. In some ways, keeping it exposed has proven beneficial, for it helps to inform others that I have a speaking difficulty. People who observe it generally try harder to listen to me, and I receive more attention, understanding, patience, and assistance.

I realized that people often gaze with interest at my filter. Young children who are more curious and less inhibited do it more often, while adults tend to be more inhibited and gaze at me when they think I am looking away.

I first encountered the curiosity of children during a trip I made to Israel. While I visited a museum near the city of Beer-Sheva I was approached by a group of young teenage Bedouin children who gathered a few feet from me, gazing and pointing at my neck. (Bedouins are Arab nomads that were recently urbanized in Israel.) My initial reaction to this open demonstration of curiosity was surprise and I was completely unprepared for such an attitude. I assumed that since they were children who lived in a desert community they had not seen anyone with such a feature and were also culturally uninhibited in showing their interest when they observed something new. One brave child actually approached me and inquired what I had; I responded by explaining to him and his friends about the nature of the filter and why I am wearing it. They accepted my explanation with great interest and some even stayed and talked with me for a while. I enjoyed talking to the children, also because I used to care for many Bedouin children during my years of pediatric residency in Israel some forty years earlier.

This incident was a fresh reminder that people are actually very interested and may be even bewildered by my neck features -these uninhibited children actually expressed what many adults truly feel.

Unfortunately, some adults exhibit what appears to be a degree of fear and worry when they see me or when they hear my cough or sneeze. I often need to cough, mainly to clear my tracheal sputum. Even though I try to avoid doing this in public, it is often unavoidable and I can not inhibit the urge to cough. I need to remove the filter from its housing very quickly before I actually cough or sneeze. I always carry a paper tissue to cover the stoma to absorb the sputum. Knowing that this may be uncomfortable for others to observe, I always try to turn my face away from others or leave the room whenever I can.

The sound of the cough is very harsh and loud. I recognize that observing me clear the stoma from secretions may be upsetting for others. Although most people are either accepting of this or are simply unable to get away from me (in a train, bus, plane or a meeting), some actually try to leave. I have encountered bus passengers or patients in doctors' offices change their seats to move away after hearing or seeing me cough. Of course this hurts my feelings, but I accept this new reality – especially since most people may not understand the nature of my problem and may worry that I have a serious medical problem that may place them at a risk of acquiring a contagious disease.

On the other hand, I have encountered acts of kindness and warmth from people I do not know. Whenever they occur, my spirits are lifted and often bring tears to my eyes. These spontaneous expressions of care are gifts that I truly cherish. They generally occur when I meet individuals who themselves have had personal experience with cancer or other serious medical problems. These individuals are obviously sensitive to these issues and are aware of how helpful their interest is.

My first such experience occurred buying tickets at a movie theatre. The ticket saleswoman spontaneously told me that she appreciated my courage and stamina in going to the theatre. She proceeded to explain that her late father was also a laryngectomee, but avoided leaving his house and interacting with people after losing his vocal chords. She enthusiastically encouraged me to continue to enjoy my life.

Another incident happened when I entered a store to purchase a mirror. The elderly saleswoman was very helpful and, before I left the store, inquired about the nature of my medical problem, pointing to my throat. I shared with her my diagnosis and why and how I had become a laryngectomee. She told me that her brother also had throat cancer, and she shared her feelings about how difficult it must be for me. Unfortunately, her brother's cancer was diagnosed too late and he died within two months. She then proceeded to tell me how she is sure that I would be okay and gave me a warm hug before I left the store.

When I had my car checked by the District of Columbia Inspection Station for the biannual emission test the inspector noted my speech difficulties and inquired if it was permanent. After I explained to him the nature of my condition he gave me a hug and blessed me with good health. His spontaneous kindness brought tears to my eyes. I did not expect such a warmth and care at that impersonal and noisy facility. The kindness of strangers always leaves me with a very warm sensation and makes me feel much better.

Most of the medical colleagues, students, and residents that I encounter on a daily basis do not talk to me about my condition. Some who I have not seen for a while politely inquire as to how I am doing. I am always heartened when some show me that they are truly interested in my situation.

Out of a group of about a dozen members of our specialty team that meets on a weekly basis only one member spontaneously inquired about my health status. When I was out of town for a few weeks she sent me an email message wondering how I was doing. When I first came back to attend our weekly meeting I immediately sensed that she was truly concerned. She genuinely inquired about my medical condition and attentively listened to my story. I learned later from her that she too had had a malignant disease and had also endured extensive surgery and treatments. That personal experience most probably made her more sensitive and appreciative of what I had endured.

A few of the residents and colleagues I work with openly asked me about my condition and showed sympathy and concern. This made me feel that people actually care about me and appreciate my presence.

I welcome people's interest and am always willing to share my medical condition with others I suspect that many individuals are actually very curious about my features but are embarrassed to ask about them. I wish more people would talk to me about my condition and allow me to break out of the shell imposed on me by my appearance and by my weak and rusty voice.

Chapter 23. Regaining My Voice

Not only was being able to speak again the greatest challenge for me, but achieving this formerly simple ability again became the most important part of my recovery. More than two years after my surgery, my weak voice remains a frustrating issue that I have slowly learned to cope with, although it is still a problem.

There are many challenges related to the rehabilitation of my voice, but the most profound difficulty has been the emotional toll. I am unable to vary my speaking tone to express emotions or alter the intensity of my voice. I can no longer audibly laugh. Although I have not cried out laud for decades, I am certain that I cannot do this as well. I find it very frustrating at times when I am unable to give voice to my happiness, anger, or frustration when I want to, and consequently, many of the emotions that I would like to express remain bottled up. I am the same person inside, yet the world no longer sees me the way I am. At times, I become angry and upset in situations where I previously could explain myself better without getting irritated.

Speaking, an effortless task before, became an elaborate and labored chore. I have to use my chest muscles and diaphragm more intensely now to force the exhaled air into the voice prosthesis. This makes talking more tiring and slow. Speaking while sitting down is more difficult than when I stand up because, in the later position, I can better use my abdominal muscles and diaphragm. My ability to speak can be interrupted suddenly and without warning by the accumulation of mucus, which I need to cough out. I can also lose my speaking ability if the HME housing that is glued to the skin breaks off and the airtight seal is thereby lost. Without a tight seal, the air I exhale escapes through the opening and does not travel into the voice prosthesis, and consequently, no voice is created when I attempt to speak.

I often find it difficult to speak when I need to. This usually happens after I have not been speaking for a while and the voice prosthesis gets plugged with mucus. It generally occurs when I wake up in the morning, and often when the phone rings. My family members became accustomed to it after some time, but it is embarrassing on occasion and creates difficulties at the most inopportune and unpredicted times.

Having a weak voice limits my ability to use my cell phone, especially out of the house and in noisy places. I can no longer respond to a call on a busy street or on the subway. Even when I use a regular phone in a quiet room, it is often difficult to hear me. This is very upsetting, especially when I call people who are not familiar with the quality of my voice. I often experience situations when others hang up when they hear me. When I called a former coworker for the first time after the surgery, he hung up the phone when he heard my voice, thinking it was a prank call. A research company that wanted to interview me over the phone declined to proceed with the interview after hearing my voice and came up with excuses to cancel it. A lawyer who had asked my advice in the past about medical malpractice issues ceased to contact me after hearing me over the phone. However, others had chosen to accept me despite my disability and continued to work with me.

When I first experienced these problems, I was very upset and hurt at other people's inability to patiently listen to me. I felt that a very important communication tool was taken away from me. I initially asked my wife to make phone calls for me, or I just avoided calling people altogether. I also resorted to using the internet and email rather than phone calls. However, I decided not to give up. I often check (and correct, if needed) my ability to speak to be sure that there is no technical problem that prevents me from responding to a phone call. I also try and make an effort to use the phone and to take care of my needs by myself whenever I have to. To increase the volume of my voice I obtained a magnification apparatus that is attached to my phone.

I also learned to immediately inform the people who talk with me over the phone about my weak voice and ask them if they have any difficulty hearing me. If they do, I request that they increase the volume of their receiver. This is helpful in some situations. Unfortunately, I still do not answer calls on my cell phone in noisy places and make phone calls less often. I am still reluctant to use my phone, and I screen incoming calls to prevent unpleasant experiences. I do not answer calls from those I do not know, and I also avoid answering calls where I do not want to share my medical condition with the callers.

It is especially difficult and challenging for me in restaurants. I try to look for quiet places and sit as close as possible to my companion. In addition to the difficulty I have with eating and speaking at the same time, it is hard for me to speak loud enough if the background noise is high. Sometimes I cannot overcome the noise to order food and have to point out my choices on the menu without speaking.

One of the frustrating aftermaths of having a very weak voice is the difficulty I experience in social gatherings where the background noise level is too high. The first time I dealt with that difficulty was when my wife and I were invited to a party that celebrated the election of President Obama. I was reluctant to accept the invitation because I could foresee the problems. I considered bringing a small microphone and speaker that I carry with me, but I have previously found that even this device does not allow me to be audible in a very noisy environment. Furthermore, carrying the microphone makes me stand out, and I feel uncomfortable. I did not want to go to the party for all the foreseeable difficulties, but I went along because I did not want to disappoint my wife.

As I predicted, the place was very noisy. The music was loud, even in places distant from the stage, and the background noise created by hundreds of people made it difficult for me to speak. My initial reaction was to stand silently by my wife and nod my head when appropriate. I then went away and sat quietly for a while. After some time, I decided to try and socialize as much as I could, but the best I could do was to whisper a few words in people's ears. This mode of communication was unsatisfactory and frustrating, and I had a feeling that others were just being polite to me and pretending to understand me out of obligation. The experience was very upsetting and disappointing. Instead of the party being a good distraction from my health problems, it made me realize that I am unable to fully participate and enjoy fun times. I was relieved when we finally left the place.

Even though my first experience in a large gathering was disappointing, I have attended parties and receptions and got accustomed to my limitations. I still find it challenging to communicate, but I found out that I can carry on a conversation and enjoy the company of others. Although it is more difficult for me to generate the loud voice needed in such a setting, it seems that I can be understood. I started to look forward to such opportunities.

An additional difficulty I have is to participate in conference calls that include multiple participants. I noted that I can be easily ignored by others, as well as the moderator, even when I try to voice my opinion or speak out. Because it is hard for other participants to hear me and since they have stronger voices, they become the dominant ones, and I am pushed to the sides and remain an outsider. I always tell the moderator ahead of time about my weak voice and request that all other participants turn the volume of their phone speaker higher. Unfortunately, others often forget to do that, although occasionally a sensitive moderator may from time to time ask me to speak.

I also find it difficult to participate in conferences and gatherings held in large rooms. I try and sit close to the podium so that I can be heard when I ask questions. I often bring a small microphone and speaker system that is of some help. In some lectures, I am assisted by the presence of a microphone that circulates among the audience at the end of the presentation so that they can ask questions. On one occasion, when there was no such microphone available, I walked over to the podium and used the speaker's microphone to ask a question. I realized that I have to be assertive and unashamed if I want to be heard.

The students I teach in medical rounds at the hospital quickly learned to listen to me attentively, and I can easily communicate with them as long as there are not too many of them and the surroundings are quiet. I have seen that when there is a group discussion and I wish to speak, the other participants yield to me even more often than they had done prior to my surgery. Some anticipate my wish to speak when I move my hand to put pressure on my HME. There are two types of HMEs: one that is hand free, which is activated by the pressure of the air in my windpipe, and another, which requires me to press it with a finger so that I can speak. Although I anticipated wanting to use a hands-free device so I could converse more naturally, I eventually preferred the manual device. Because this method requires me to place a finger over the HME, it signals to others that I wish to speak. The social cue became just as important as the HME device itself.

However, speaking in these settings is not as smooth as I wish it would be and is often a source of frustration. In some of the meetings that I regularly attend, the participants are very vocal and competitive and strive to speak as much as possible, filling up all the allotted time. In these settings, I often find myself pushed aside and ignored. I realized that I have to assert myself and compete for my place if I want to be heard. On one occasion, I became more and more frustrated and upset as I felt ignored by everyone, even though I tried to signal my wishes to speak. As I kept failing to be noticed, the level of my frustration grew to the point that I even wanted to leave the room as a sign of protest. I finally decided to speak up by interrupting the discussion and told the participants that I also wish to speak and because of my weak voice I want them to pay more attention to me whenever I signaled I want to speak. This assertive and direct approach was new for me but it seemed to work. Since this incident, I noticed a change in the attitude of the participants and, even though I sometimes need to wait for my turn to speak, this group has become more attentive to my needs.

I occasionally encounter difficulties with other people accepting my weak voice; sometimes it seems to border on overt discrimination. An example was the attitude I faced when I responded to an invitation to participate in a medical survey about treatment options for pneumonia with a new antibiotic. The survey was conducted by a medical research company for which I had previously consulted.

Upon my arrival in their office for the first time after my surgery, I was directed by the receptionist to a waiting area. After about ten minutes a junior staff member walked in and asked me if I would need anything to speak better. Before I could respond to his question, he abruptly left the room mumbling that he would return shortly. He obviously did not know how to react to my visible HME and rusty voice. After an additional ten minutes the company's director walked in and told me that he wondered if my interviewer would have trouble listening to me and recording the dialogue. I assured him that I can be heard very well in a small room and that they would have no trouble recording the interview. After an additional ten minutes the interviewer came in to see and hear me for himself and again questioned if I could be heard well.

I was ready to throw in the towel and leave, but decided not to let my weak voice stand in my way. I was not going to be pushed aside just because I had a disability. I assured the interviewer that the interview would work out, as I had no trouble speaking. The one hour discussion was flawless and, even though I spoke slower than I had in the past, the interviewers realized that my opinions and vast experience could be an important resource of information and advice.

I was happy a few months later to be invited again by the same company to participate in a new medical survey. It made me feel good that my weak voice was not an impediment to be asked again. To my surprise, I encountered the same questions from both the receptionist and the company's director evidencing doubt about my ability to speak. Even though they obviously knew and remembered me, they again asked whether I could participate in the interview. As I did previously, I completed this interview successfully. However, this experience was an acute reminder that I may always face a harsh reality of potential discrimination based on the quality of my voice.

Another consequence of having a weak voice is its impact on my lecturing ability. Prior to the laryngectomy, I was a very popular and effective public speaker. I gave numerous lectures across the country and overseas. However, the laryngectomy changed this completely. Even though I had given many local, national, and even international lectures, I was frustrated by the difficulties I now have in delivering these talks. I always need a microphone, speak slower than before, and lecturing is more difficult for me now because of the increased effort I have in producing a sound. I wonder if I will ever be invited to lecture again by those who had actually heard me. So far, I have not received a repeat invitation by an organization to speak again after delivering a lecture with my new voice.

I am always terrified at the possibility that the seal around my stoma will break in the middle of my lecture and I will be embarrassed in front of the audience because I will not be able to continue. Fortunately, that has not happened yet. To prevent it, I use a larger base for my HME and glue it very firmly a short time prior to my talk.

Some of the invitations I still get are from organizations that are not aware of my handicap. Prior to writing this book and publishing articles about my surgery, I did not share my personal medical status widely. Accepting these speaking assignments and actually delivering the lectures constitute a personal challenge and subsequently an accomplishment for me. When I am successful, it lifts my self-confidence and enhances my recovery. However, this is always mixed with frustration because I know that I am not as good a speaker as I used to be.

My experiences in speaking in public again were one of the major issues I dealt with. Returning to the speaker's podium and finding the right audience was a great challenge I had to overcome.

Chapter 24. Back at the Speaker's Podium

My first experience giving a lecture took place only ten weeks after my laryngectomy. I was to lecture to an audience of about 150 family practitioners at an annual meeting of a state medical society. This was a major endeavor for me, as I had not yet traveled by air or stayed in a hotel after the surgery. Prior to the surgery, I loved to travel. Sometimes I spent more than a month a year on the road. But now, after my surgery, simple travel was fraught with difficulty. I was worried that I would not be able to bring all my medical supplies in my carry-on luggage and that I might develop problems breathing the dry air in the airplane.

I wanted to give the talk and succeed in my presentation at all costs. However, prior to accepting the invitation to give the talk, I wanted to make sure that I could actually deliver the lecture. I practiced in front of a mirror at home. Then, at the university where I teach, I tested my ability to speak and be heard in a large auditorium using a microphone. It was only after proving to myself that I could actually present the lecture successfully that I accepted the assignment. I informed the manager of the continued medical education (CME) organization that invited me that I had had surgery and that my voice was weak but assured him that it projects well when I use a microphone. He accepted the news without posing any questions or concerns. I had been invited by this manger to give CME lectures numerous times in the previous ten years, so I felt we had a good working relationship.

The travel by plane and car was uneventful, and I was happy to find out that I was able to manage my breathing and voice prosthesis well on the road. Even though I had delivered thousands of lectures, I was nervous and apprehensive before this talk. A few months earlier, the word "talk" or "lecture" was something I was unsure I could ever do again.

When I arrived at the conference center, I was greeted by the manager of the inviting CME organization. This was the first time that he saw me after the surgery, and he did not hide his surprise and immediately voiced his concerns about my ability to deliver the lecture. I reassured him that I was able to do it adequately.

I started my lecture by letting the audience know about my current condition and how special this talk was for me because it was the first one after my surgery. I decided that it was best to inform the audience about my condition so that they did not wonder why I speak the way I do and also to prepare them for the possibility that my voice might fail me or would be difficult to understand. I did this in all my future presentations, and it made me feel more at ease. I gave the talk to the best of my abilities, and the audience was very attentive and asked me numerous questions. Only a handful of listeners left the auditorium during my talk, and I was applauded for almost a minute.

Giving the lecture was not easy. At times, my voice became weak, and I realized that because of my stiff neck muscles, I did not have the ability to move my head back and forth from the audience to the screen. I had to find a standing position that allowed me to generate a strong voice while facing the audience and viewing the screen. This was difficult at times, and I finally gave up on moving my neck and shifted my whole body instead. I also had to pause a few times to catch my breath and had to slow down the speed of my speech. However, I had a wonderful feeling of accomplishment at the end of my talk and knew that I had come over a major barrier on the way to recovery.

At the end of my talk I did not get any feedback about the quality of my performance from the manager of the CME program. He only asked me if my voice would improve overtime, to which I answered that I hope that it is going to get better, but it will never be similar to the one I had before. Since I had to leave immediately after my talk and there was no intermission between my talk and the next one, I had no chance to speak to any of the attendees and was therefore not sure how well my talk was received. Even though I felt that I did an adequate job, I was unsure and was yearning for feedback. A few weeks later, I corresponded with the manger of the CME organization inquiring about the results of the audience's evaluation of my performance.

His response was, "Attached is the data from your lecture. I thought you did an admirable job. I just wish you would've been up front about your voice... you kinda blindsided me." It was clear to me that he was unhappy with my performance and thought that I should have told him more about my situation before my lecture.

The audience evaluation was "excellent" by 67 percent of the participants, "average" by 27 percent, and "poor" by 4 percent. I felt good about such evaluation, and told him that I was happy to see the very positive evaluations I received. He dimmed my enthusiasm bluntly by stating, "In comparing the evaluation you received to other speakers, I wouldn't necessarily call them positive. I don't say that to discourage you, just to give you constructive feedback."

This manager did not invite me to give a lecture again. I feel hurt by this rejection, especially since I had given numerous lectures for that CME program since its inception. It represents the cruel reality that after suffering the irreversible loss of my natural voice, I was no longer of any use to the program. I rationalized his decision by his wish to use speakers who can deliver a lecture in a natural voice because they are evidently better presenters. I was disappointed by his lack of loyalty to me and his inability to see how inspirational my talk could be to physicians who can see a rehabilitated person.

An example of this harsh reality was my experience with another CME organization with whom I have also worked for many years. When one of their mangers called me to discuss future programs he was astounded by my weak and rusty voice. It took him a minute to continue the conversation and I felt he was unsure how to proceed after I explained the nature of my voice. He ended the conversation abruptly and promised to call me back but never did. I have not heard from his organization again.

One of my most challenging presentations was to deliver a lecture about upper respiratory infections at the Annual Turkish National Pediatric Congress. This was a major endeavor for me eight months after the surgery because I had to fly overseas for the first time. This trip involved taking six flights and flying over 4,500 miles. A few weeks before the scheduled talk, the sponsors learned about my surgery from one of the local otolaryngologists. I had contacted this specialist in my efforts to find a local speech pathologist in case I needed one during my visit. They questioned my ability to speak, but I assured them that I performed well giving lectures as long as I have a microphone. I very much wanted to succeed in my presentation and practiced it several times before giving it.

The lecture in Turkey was for about 250 physicians, and since more than two-thirds of them listened through simultaneous translation, I was less concerned that they would not be able to understand me. I was, however, apprehensive about failing to deliver an adequate presentation at a national meeting and disappointing my hosts. I was concerned about the audience's reactions to my voice when they actually heard me. I have lectured in Turkey many times before and had a reputation there I did not want to spoil.

When I landed in Turkey and was met by my hosts, I was wondering if they were disappointed at the quality of my voice. Even though everyone was very pleasant and friendly to me, I was unable to know what they actually thought. I kept wondering if the organizers regretted asking me to give the lecture. I felt too uncomfortable to ask them directly after my talk how well I did, but judging by the audience's attentiveness, I felt I did well. I was reassured by the fact that only a few of listeners left the lecture hall during my talk, and I had numerous follow-up questions. Several clinicians approach me after my presentation with more questions, and many expressed their gratitude for the information they gained. Despite all of this, I had lingering doubts because I compared myself to the way I was able to deliver a talk before my surgeries. I was, however, very gratified to be able to deliver my talk and for the audience appreciation. This was a major accomplishment for me and reinforced my sense of wellbeing and independence.

Following that lecture, I flew to Israel where I visited family and friends and also gave two lectures in Hebrew. They were given in major medical centers to small groups of specialists. I was less nervous lecturing in Israel because my talks were in smaller venues, and many members in the audience were my friends. I was surprised to see a familiar face in one of my lectures that I had not seen in twenty-five years – my high school mentor, who had introduced me to microbiology when I was sixteen years old and thereby sparked my love of science. He had retired several years ago after heading the department of microbiology at one of the local medical schools and came especially to hear my lecture. I was touched that I could rekindle our friendship and demonstrate to him my appreciation for his mentorship.

One important presentation I had was in Oxford England for an annual course given to physicians from many countries about infections in children. I was asked to speak on a topic about which I am a known expert and I have long had personal relationships with many of the speakers. Unlike my previous lectures, where I felt uncomfortable revealing the full extent of my surgeries, one of the organizers was a good friend and former student who knew all about my speaking difficulties. I was, however, apprehensive about delivering a lecture at such a prestigious place and to people who mattered to me. When I arrived in Oxford and met the organizers, I re-experienced the familiar uncertainty of wondering whether they were disappointed to hear my weak voice and whether they doubted my ability to give the lecture. Even though they did not challenge me, I felt the need to bring the topic up and assured them that I was confident that my delivery of the lecture would be adequate.

I started my presentation by explaining to the audience that I speak without vocal cords and even explained how my voice is generated. I wanted the participants to understand why I speak the way I do, not to gain their sympathy. To my surprise, they responded by applauding me for quite some time. I presented a talk that I had given before, but because I spoke at a slower pace, I used only about half of the slides and economized with my words, using the most effective ones. I employed the techniques I had always used and looked into the eyes of each of the over 200 attendees. They were very attentive, and many nodded their heads in response to my explanations as if to signal me that they understood or agreed with me. I felt very connected to them. At the end of my talk, I fielded numerous questions, and many participants came to ask for more details. For the first time since my surgery, a few people even told me how much they enjoyed my talk.

As in previous lectures, I was not convinced that I did a good enough job. In my mind, I could picture and hear the way I used to speak and wished I could still speak the same way. It made me envious of the other speakers who could speak much faster and deliver more information. When I confessed my doubts to one of the attendees, he responded by saying, "but you were so concise and to the point and delivered what we really need to know, and I remember what you have said much better than what others did, partially because they said so many unnecessary things." It was good to hear it, but in my gut I doubted how genuine people were to my face. I suspected that I was told encouraging things because they felt sorry for me.

I felt a little better when some of the organizers and speakers emailed me their responses after I had sent them a recent paper I had published in *The Journal of the American Medical Association* about rediscovering my voice. Here is some of what they wrote:

"I think we all felt rather privileged to hear you speak in Oxford, and I am delighted that you were able to stand up and do so and share your knowledge with the audience."

"Your words are very inspiring, as was your talk in Oxford. We were all so touched and unsure whether we could have ourselves made such progress. It must have been utterly exhausting."

"I must say that I was impressed that your voice did not limit your ability to present a very successful teaching session at our recent meeting in Oxford. I, for one, very much look forward to hearing you speak at the next opportunity."

"Please let me express my deep admiration for your determination and will to continue your great career as a worldwide known pediatric infectious diseases specialist and THE expert in anaerobic infections despite your recent surgery. It was an inspiration for me, and I am convinced that the audience shared my feelings."

"It was good to be with you at Oxford, but it was unexpected and surprising to learn of your cancer and radical surgical procedures. Now that you have sent us the piece submitted to the JAMA, we can only admire further your willingness to participate in a meeting such as the infectious disease symposium there and the physical and emotional obstacles you have overcome so successfully. Truly, you have served as an inspiration to all of us."

"I greatly enjoyed your lecture in Oxford, and I admire the way you have overcome the challenges caused by the laryngectomy and the subsequent inability to speak. Thanks again on behalf of many in the audience and specifically my Dutch colleagues. I wish you all the best and hope to meet again in the future!"

After receiving these encouraging messages, I started to believe that I can still give a powerful lecture and the audience actually can learn from me.

In all of my speeches after my surgery, I struggled with the feeling that I was an inadequate public speaker. However, one lecture changed my idea who my audience should be. Six months after my surgery, I was to deliver a lecture at the Annual Meeting of the

American Academy of Otolaryngology-Head and Neck Surgery that took place in Chicago. I was to speak about tonsillar infections, an area about which I had done substantial research. I wanted to fulfill my commitment to give that lecture, especially since it was the first time I was asked to speak at that prestigious meeting. I also hoped that some of the surgeons who operated on me would be able to attend my presentation. I wanted them to see how far I had come. I also knew that an audience of otolaryngologists would be more receptive and appreciative of my speaking efforts.

My lecture was part of a symposium. In preparation, the chairman organized several phone conferences with the speakers. I had great difficulty speaking up during those conferences. The other participants in these phone conferences were all established and renowned otolaryngologists. To my surprise, they displayed a lack of collegial decorum by ignoring my attempts to speak out, even though the chairperson informed them about my condition in advance. He was gracious to ask me to give my input, and when I shared with him my apprehensions about my ability to perform well, he assured me that I would be addressing an audience that would understand of my condition.

Presenting that lecture was very challenging. In attendance were about 120 participants and, in the audience, I saw someone I recognized from the crew that cared for me after my laryngectomy. One of the residents who took care of me had come to hear my lecture, although he did not know in advance that I would be speaking. It was rewarding to speak to him afterwards, something I could not do at the hospital when we first met. I was also happy to meet in person one of the specialists who advised me by email and phone about my surgical choices and thanked him personally for it. It was also an opportunity to meet some colleagues and discuss their research.

When my talk was over, it dawned on me for the first time that I will never be able to perform as well as I did before. I was envious of the speakers before and after me for having clear and brisk voices. I missed my old voice, and even though I did the best I could, I could not measure up to the quality of the other speakers.

I realized that instead of struggling to compare myself with other speakers and with my past abilities, I needed to find a place where my rusty voice would be appreciated. I had to accept that I would no longer be as popular a speaker as I had been before the laryngectomy. The fact is that, given the choice, organizers will select other individuals who do not have any speaking impairment or deficiencies. The only topics where the organizers may be willing to accept my disability and ask me to lecture are those about which I am the best expert.

It occurred to me at that moment that there is one area where my impaired speech may be an advantage rather than a weakness. This is when I speak about my challenges dealing with cancer and direct my lecture to health care providers specializing in that area as well as laryngectomees.

As I looked around the convention hall, I also realized that I was in a unique venue for making some contacts with organizations and companies that could help me achieve that goal. I visited the exhibition hall and introduced myself to the companies that produce and distribute the products used for speech in patients after laryngectomy. Unlike my previous experience dealing with pharmaceutical companies producing antibiotics, the products displayed in the booths were not for someone else – they were for me. I was using those medical devices to speak to their producers. I was fortunate to meet with the presidents and senior officers of these companies, and I established contacts which later enhanced my abilities to reach out to many laryngectomees clubs throughout the country. I was also able to initiate a research project to evaluate a new filter system that can reduce the rate of respiratory infections in laryngectomees.

On the way to the airport to fly back home, I realized that I had just opened a new avenue for myself that could impact my life in a very significant and positive way.

The realization that my best audiences are fellow patients and their care givers was reinforced following my presentation of Grand Rounds in Otolaryngology in the university hospital where I teach. I was asked by the head of the department to present my personal experience as a patient who had had a laryngectomy. It was the first opportunity I had to tell my own story to otolaryngologists who care for patients like me. The applause I received at the end of my talk was not for the quality of my voice, but for the content of my words. I was not judging myself against the previous lectures I had given, because I gave an entirely new talk based on my pre and post-surgical experiences. After the forty-five-minute talk, several of the residents and staff members told me how appreciative they were of the lecture. In fact, they told me that my presentation would change their approach to their own patients because they had gained a better understanding of the illness and its treatment through the eyes of the patient. After hearing my honest input, some critical and some appreciative of my care, they felt that they were better equipped to deal with their patients.

Following my presentation, one of the staff members initiated a request to the American Academy of Otolaryngology-Head and Neck Surgery to invite me to deliver such a talk at their next Annual Meeting.

When the talk ended, I realized that I found an important venue by which my personal suffering and difficulties could be turned into something positive. I discovered how to change my lemon into lemonade.

Epilogue. Finding a New Mission

I have always needed a purpose and a positive goal in my life. This keeps me going forward and helps me overcome difficult times. After retiring and losing the voice I was born with, I searched for a new target and mission in life. I wanted to prevent myself from sliding into depression and desperation and yearned to find a purpose that would not only help me, but serve others as well. A part of me was very pessimistic and only saw a downhill road ahead with no hope in sight.

I was fortunate to find a new direction to avoid the chasm of a purposeless life. This occurred unexpectedly during a family event, where I met an oral surgeon who was a brain cancer survivor. He told me how he was able to find a new purpose and meaning to his life by talking to and helping other cancer patients. He also rediscovered his love of building ship models using his handcraft skills. He seemed to have found a new avenue to express his talents and use his own experiences with cancer to uplift the spirits of others. He urged me to also find a new meaning and direction. His optimism and enthusiasm were infectious and affected me deeply. I feel fortunate to have met him at a critical period of my life when I could have slid into depression. I followed his advice and began walking down a new road.

I decided to start writing down my experiences in a series of articles for otolaryngologists and other health care providers as well as laryngectomees. I thought that this will benefit others who had undergone similar experiences and open the eyes of health care providers to the feelings and tribulations of their patients. I first wrote a short manuscript entitled "Neck Cancer- A Physicians' Personal Experience" for the *Archives of Otolaryngology Head and Neck Surgery,* a major otolaryngology journal about my physical and emotional journey as a patient who had a laryngectomy. I addressed the errors that were made in my care, and the need for greater personal attention to, as well as support and compassion for, patients who undergo laryngectomy as well as the hardship and struggles that follow the surgery. I also expressed gratitude to all of my care givers who did their best to cure me from cancer and save my life. One reviewer of the manuscript requested that I delete the description of the mistakes that were made during my care because they "do not fit the rest of the story." I reluctantly did this so that the manuscript could be accepted for publication but felt that by doing so a unique opportunity was missed to get the attention of surgeons so that future mistakes could be avoided.

Once the paper was published I received numerous messages from otolaryngologists, other clinicians and SLPs, as well as laryngectomees who appreciated my input. Many health care professionals told me that reading about my experiences opened their eyes and made them appreciate the difficulties that patients experiences. Several told me that this manuscript should be read by all medical students and physicians in training. Some of the responses were very revealing and touching and showed me that there were many wonderful and sensitive caregivers who genuinely strive to help laryngectomees.

A few of these responses:

"I am a speech pathologist in Arizona and I work with a large population of patients with oral, head and neck cancer. Much of what I do is with the laryngectomy population. I am also the co-facilitator for our local chapter of SPOHNC (Support for People with Oral, Head and Neck Cancer). Your words are so very true. I strive to be the type of health care professional that is there for my patients to provide education, encouragement, and compassion.

Thank you for the reminders. I hope that the others within the intended audience will be receptive to your suggestions. Thank you for sharing your story."

"Thank you for sharing your article. I will be making copies and I will have them available to the SPOHNC support group. What you describe as your personal experience is heard over and over again. I am continually astounded at the rush to treat with little to no attention given to the work of healing. Patients and their support are left to fend with very little direction, teaching, or involvement unless it is to 'another appointment' to someone with little connection to the situation and another large bill, that insurance may not honor. With head and neck cancer survivors, the treatment is tremendous and the recovery is long term with new side-effects appearing after time has passed from treatment. Yet, I am always amazed by what I hear. For example, a survivor in my group had bilateral neck radiation with fields extending to the mid-face and never was told to see a dentist before treatment. Imagine how he felt when his teeth began to crumble and he learned that a dentist visit is a standard recommendation prior to radiation. Let alone the cost of hyperbaric treatments that he had and the constant fear of osteoradionecrosis he has. Let alone the anger he feels that such a simple preemptive treatment of fluoride trays might have prevented this problem. The survivors' stories go on and on."

"I do so wish that there would be a 'revolution' (so to speak) in our healthcare system to return to the value of compassion and truly caring for our fellow man. As a nurse for over thirty years, I am saddened to see the how focus of the bottom line now undermines the very essence of good care. I believe that listening, touching, observing... communicating... (Hence assessing and teaching) with the patient has as much importance as modern technology; perhaps more so because of technology. As a registered nurse, my training is to be a team member with the physician to address these very issues. However, our role is now shaped (misshaped) by the 'bottom-line'. I have seen a deterioration of healthcare at such an alarming speed and no money thrown at it will improve it. The very caring that you ascribe to must come from the core of those involved in caring for the infirm enough to say stop and to return to the essence of health CARE."

"Your editorial certainly touched me I wish you the very best. Thank you for caring enough to share and I do hope that many will listen."

"Your article is extremely well-written and very much needed. While many clinicians who treat this patient population are compassionate, there is still much for professionals to learn when dealing with patients who have speaking and other problems related to treatment. Your article should be required reading for every head and neck clinician (especially the incoming Residents and Fellows!). I run a support group in Boston (a chapter of SPOHNC). I will make sure to share this with all of my group members, some of whom are physicians. Thank you again for this excellent article!"

"I am very moved by your article and will gladly forward it within our Department of Radiation Medicine. I will also share it with members of our
support group. Thank you so much for sharing!"

A synopsis of the paper was also published in the monthly newsletter of the International Association of Laryngectomees, who also invited me to speak and participate in several workshops and discussion panels at their annual meeting. I also heard from several laryngectomee clubs across the country who wished to distribute my paper among their members, and several of them also invited me to speak at their monthly and regional annual meetings.

The second short manuscript was called "Rediscovering My Voice" and describes the difficulties I had in speaking and lecturing and how I found a new audience when I spoke about my experiences as a laryngectomee. This paper was published a few months later in the Journal of the American Medical Association (JAMA). After its publication I received over 150 messages from medical professionals as well as laryngectomees who were very inspired and moved by the manuscript.

Some of the messages:

"I truly enjoyed your narrative in JAMA. As a medical student, your story reinforces the 'why' of medicine. Whether a person is a therapist, nurse, janitor or doctor, we are there for the totality of a human being who happens to be a patient. Your story reminds me of a quote, 'The best way to care for the patient is to care about the patient.'"

"I just completed reading your published article. Hopefully, doctors and other professionals will have a greater understanding of our situation. Keep up your enlightening articles."

"Congratulations on having your article accepted by JAMA. I'm sure a lot of physicians will benefit from reading it and understand laryngectomee life now in a way they could not relate to before."

"I was very moved by your experience, and how you turned a terribly difficult situation into an opportunity to do good for many. Thank you for having the courage to share your experience and for the good work you have done, and continue to do."

"Excellent article. I'm constantly amazed how people have adjusted to their new lives. What strikes me most is they find a strength and confidence that before their surgery they would have not thought they possessed."

"Thanks for sharing and not giving up. You are an inspiration - keep up the good work."

"From the heart! Well done!! Do keep that positive approach to your life's activities."

"Thank you for your article... Unless you are a lary, you do not know how other lary's feel. Doctors need to present the mental side of losing your voice and not just the physical side... and they need to show compassion. They have to realize that a person's life is forever changed with the loss of their voice... they almost lose their identity. It takes a strong person to overcome such adversity."

"I found the article to be an extremely moving and inspirational piece that is sure to have an impact on anyone who reads it."

"You've been through a great deal, and I think that your efforts to share your experiences with others is phenomenal."

"Your article was wonderful. A very important lesson for me. I was a teacher for seventeen years and enjoyed – no, loved - the audience's reaction to my presentations. But now I am a lary, (one year) unable to speak except with a 'buzzing' electronic device which is unsuitable for an audience. I have been told and encouraged to get a voice prosthesis installed, but I am still not convinced that it would have a positive effect on my voice clarity. Your advice would be very appreciated. Thank you very much."

"Thank you for sharing an inspiring real life story. I'm forwarding your story on to the members of my support group. We all have had life changing experiences due to oral head and neck cancer and appreciate what challenges you have gone through. You are an inspiration to others."

"I just read your words. I could not wait to let you know how inspired I was by your expression."

"This was a very moving and touching piece. You have taken your illness and given it meaning and purpose for the greater good. Hope you remain on the path of good health."

"Your words speak much louder than your voice. Please share your experiences with every medical student with whom you have contact. I admire your courage. Keep TALKING the good talk."

"I just read your article, and was deeply touched. You are so courageous, but then you have just demonstrated in another way your incredible spirit and passion for passing on what you have learned and experienced so others could learn from you."

"The story of your amazing rehabilitation is indeed exciting! We hope that you will carry on with your very unique mission"

"This was great. Printed it for my students and speech pathologists to read!"

"As a physician who was just diagnosed with papillary thyroid carcinoma and recently underwent a modified radical neck dissection and thyroidectomy, I can appreciate your point of view 'on the other side'. Reading your article in JAMA was encouraging and uplifting. You truly have found some meaning and purpose in something that otherwise seems random and pointless like cancer. I applaud your efforts but more importantly wish you a continued speedy recovery, improvement and continued good health. Thank you again for your selflessness in writing about your story and sharing it with others."

"Your article, 'Rediscovering My Voice,' was fabulous. Very moving and I am sure your fellow laryngopharyngectomees are appreciative of a physician understanding everything they are experiencing."

"Your article was terrific! You conveyed so much with your writing... your struggle, your feelings, and your adaptation to such a difficult illness and treatment. I am glad that, although the cancer took your normal speaking voice, it did not take your intellect, compassion or empathy."

The third manuscript I prepared was longer and described in detail the medical and surgical treatment I received, the medical errors that were made, and the emotional and physical difficulties that I had to struggle with. I felt that it should be read by the specialists who care for patients with head and neck cancer. However, my attempts to get the paper accepted for publication in one of the major otolaryngological journals in the USA failed. The reason given for the rejections by most journals is that they did not have a section devoted to manuscripts about personal experiences. I also wondered if my honest criticism of the surgeons who took care of me contributed to the rejection. The paper was finally published in *Surgical Oncology* a medical journal devoted to cancer surgery.

One reader wrote:

"I just thought you would like to know that 'A Physician's Experience as a Cancer of the Neck Patient' published in *Surgical Oncology* was chosen as one of the articles to be discussed at our next journal club. I am a senior resident in ENT at Montreal University and appreciate you sharing your personal journey from a physician's perspective. I hope to be able to inspire and bring more awareness to our medical team regarding your experience."

I also became very involved in responding to inquiries by fellow laryngectomees that were posted in the daily internet newsletter, WebWhispers.com. This site allows laryngectomees to share their experiences and to assist each other in medical and other problems. It was and still is an invaluable resource for me at difficult times and I was glad that I could reciprocate and assist others who had problems about which I could provide some guidance. I only respond to questions if I feel knowledgeable enough and had personal experience in the topic. My advice is based on my medical knowledge as well as on my personal experiences and provides possible solutions for dealing with these problems.

I responded to questions such as the effects of radiation on dental health, the development of local and systemic infections, the nervous system, blood pressure issues, and eating and thyroid gland function problems. I also share with others practical details of how I achieved the ability to seal my HME housing and clean my voice prosthesis. I always encourage others to seek direct medical care and not only rely on my advice.

I had my first opportunity to meet with and speak to fellow laryngectomees when I was invited to deliver a lecture about my personal experiences and rehabilitation at the combined annual meeting of International Society of Laryngectomees and the Voice Institute fifteen months after my surgery. The more than two hundred attendees were laryngectomees like myself who came from all over the world. During the meeting they attended seminars and symposiums by experienced SLPs and other experts and received practical advice on improving their speaking abilities. I was fortunate to finally meet Dr. Mark Singer, the co-inventor of the voice prosthesis that enables me to speak. His lecture gave a historical perspective on the means by which laryngectomees were able to speak in the past and how the development of the voice prosthesis made it much easier. I felt fortunate to be able to benefit from his invention. After his lecture he offered me some practical advice, such as how to position my neck when speaking, which improved the quality of my voice.

I also participated on a medical panel that responded to audience questions about their medical problems. I was happy to be able to help others by sharing my personal experiences and solutions to problems. For example, one person asked about the difficulties he had in maintaining a good seal around the base that holds his HME. There were many questions about the emotional hardships and struggles in adjusting to life as a laryngectomee. For example, one man wondered how to deal with the uncertainty of the future after the diagnosis of cancer and the depression that follows.

I shared with the audience my personal difficulties and struggles and the way I finally overcame them. I gave the audience tips about improving the practical skills of dealing with the daily maintenance of their prosthesis and airways and explained the reasons why medical difficulties exist and how they can be overcome. It was enlightening to see how I could help others with the insights I had gained in such a short period of time. After one of my responses, I received spontaneous applause. It meant a lot to me to hear it.

My lecture about my experiences during and after the surgeries was also well received, and some of the attendees came up to thank me. One person told me that she was moved to tears by some of what I said. In a surprising moment, a man from Texas told me he relived his own experience with cancer while he was listening to my talk. I felt that I was finally able to see others benefit from my experiences. Most importantly, I felt a strong camaraderie with new friends and acquaintances who share my plight.

I was fortunate to have more opportunities to speak about my personal experiences to other laryngectomee groups, as well as to the otolaryngologists who care for them. In my lectures, I speak about facing and living through the difficulties and tribulations of post-laryngectomy life. I recount how dependent and helpless I became after that surgery. I describe how it feels being unable to speak, eat, and breathe normally while dealing with a potential fatal illness. This new reality made me extremely vulnerable both physically and emotionally. I stress how in this difficult and challenging time, health care providers need to appreciate what their patients are feeling. I remain more convinced than ever that it is the duty of doctors, nurses, and SLPs to provide competent and compassionate care to help their patients endure a very challenging period of their lives.

I offer suggestions how to improve the patient's post-surgical care. I stress the need to educate the patients and their families prior to their surgeries about the short and long-term medical and social implications of the procedures they are about to have. For the surgical team, I suggest that they spend more time with individual patients and better communicate with them during a period when their world changes dramatically and they actually realize that they are unable to speak. Patients need to be constantly informed and involved in their medical care and understand their changing condition. Surgeons need to appreciate how overwhelming is the realization that one's vocal cords are gone forever.

I also advocate implementing standard techniques by nursing care and greater vigilance and better communication among staff to avoid medical errors. Nurses and other health care personnel have to be sensitive to the special needs of laryngectomees who can not verbalize their thoughts and requirements. I stress why surgeons in training should be educated about the proper medical and psychological post-surgical care and the special requirement of patients after major surgery, including laryngectomy.

I was especially gratified to be able to assist Dr. Marker, the surgeon who performed my laryngectomy, in his efforts to educate the public in the early detection of head and neck cancer. A foundation which Dr. Marker created organized a free oral cancer screening for the New York City area in an effort to generate public awareness and encourage individuals to seek medical help so that their cancer can be discovered early. I wrote a short article about my "patient story" which was used as an example of how early detection is critical and how, despite losing my vocal cords, I was able to return to useful and productive life. My personal story of speaking again in public

267

helped make throat cancer more real. The concept was promoted in the local media and achieved a wide ranging community outreach that brought in many patients for test screenings. Such screenings are especially important for individuals who have been smoking for many years and those who have any symptoms of persistent throat pain, difficulty in swallowing, or have a change in their voice such as hoarseness.

My wish is to use this obstacle in my life in a positive way. By lecturing and writing about my experiences and sharing them with other laryngectomees and health care providers, I hope that others will learn and benefit from my experience. Speaking about my experiences opened an avenue for me for share them with caregivers in the hope that they better understand and appreciate how their patients feel during such a life altering diagnosis and surgery. I hope they will be able to help their patients confront cancer by improving their clinical approach with a more humane touch. Likewise, I hope that laryngectomees can benefit from my personal experiences and practical advice and realize that their own experiences, feelings, and responses are shared by others.

My ability to speak – even with a rusty and weak voice – becomes an asset in these settings rather than a liability. I can serve as a symbol of recovery and set an example of resilience to other patients. My speech also provides health care providers with a sense of accomplishment. I was also a patient and, therefore, my progress illustrates that their skills in saving patients' lives and in reconstructing their airways have a positive result. I wanted to show other patients that we can remain active and that we can regain our previous speaking abilities, even without vocal cords.

I obviously cannot perform in the same way as a speaker with their vocal cords intact. However, I have found a new meaning in my life that helps me as well as others. I hope that I can use this unexpected obstacle in my life in a positive way. Most importantly, I have realized that my present voice can be an asset rather than a handicap.

This book is an outgrowth of those lectures, and writing it is part of my recovery. I hope that it will assist others in dealing with trying times in their own lives. For those professionals who are helping us to heal, I hope the book will shed some insight into the struggles and challenges that we patients with cancer of the head and neck face and how we strive to overcome them. Hopefully, it will lead them to better understand and deal diligently and compassionately with their patients.

###

2/2013

Made in the USA
Charleston, SC
20 May 2012